Internet fo
Nursing Research

A Guide to Strategies, Skills,
and Resources

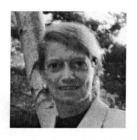

Joyce J. Fitzpatrick, PhD, MBA, RN, FAAN, is the Elizabeth Brooks Ford Professor of Nursing, Frances Payne Bolton School of Nursing, Case Western Reserve University (CWRU) in Cleveland, Ohio, where she was Dean from 1982 through 1997. She has received numerous honors and awards including the *American Journal of Nursing* Book of the Year Award 18 times. Dr. Fitzpatrick is widely published in nursing and health care literature. She is senior editor of the *Annual Review of Nursing Research* series, now in its 21st volume, and editor of the National League for Nursing journal, *Nursing Education Perspectives*. In 1998 Dr. Fitzpatrick edited the classic *Encyclopedia of Nursing Research* and a series of Research Digests, including *Nursing Research Digest, Maternal Child Health Nursing Research Digest, Geriatric Nursing Research Digest,* and *Psychiatric Mental Health Nursing Research Digest.* She has coedited three recent books focused on nurses and the internet: *Internet Resources for Nurses* (2000), *Nurses Guide to Consumer Health Web Sites* (2001), and *Essentials of Internet Use for Nurses* (2002).

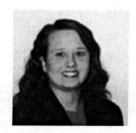

Kristen S. Montgomery, PhD, RN, is an Assistant Professor at the University of South Carolina College of Nursing. She received her doctorate in nursing from the Frances Payne Bolton School of Nursing, Case Western Reserve University, Cleveland, Ohio. She earned her MSN from the University of Pennsylvania, in Philadelphia, Pennsylvania and her BSN from Oakland University in Rochester, Michigan. Dr. Montgomery completed a postdoctoral research fellowship in health promotion and risk reduction at the University of Michigan School of Nursing in Ann Arbor. Dr. Montgomery's program of research is focused on improving birth outcomes among high-risk pregnant populations. She has coedited four other books, two of the them focused on Internet use among nurses.

Internet for Nursing Research

A Guide to Strategies, Skills, and Resources

Joyce J. Fitzpatrick, PhD, RN, FAAN
Kristen S. Montgomery, PhD, RN

Editors

Springer Publishing Company

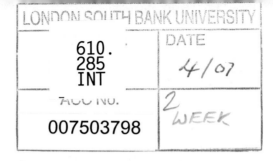
Springer Publishing Company, Inc.
11 West 42nd Street
New York, NY 10036

Aquisitions Editor: Ruth Chasek
Production Editor: Sara Yoo
Cover design by Joanne E. Honigman

04 05 06 07 08 / 5 4 3 2 1

Library of Congress Cataloging-in-Publication Data

Internet for nursing research : a guide to strategies, skills, and resources / Joyce J. Fitzpatrick and Kristen S. Montgomery, editors.
    p. cm.
  Includes bibliographical references and index.
  ISBN 0-8261-4545-0
  1. Nursing—Research—Computer network resources. 2. Nursing—Research—Data processing. 3. Nursing informatics. 4. Internet.
  [DNLM: 1. Nursing Research—methods. 2. Data Collection—methods. 3. Information Systems. 4. Internet. 5. Nursing Research—education.
WY 20.5 I619   2004] I. Fitzpatrick, Joyce J., 1944– II. Montgomery, Kristen S.
  RT81.5.I58   2004
  610'.285—dc22   2004016646

Printed in the United States of America by IBT Global.

Contents

Part III: Teaching Research Online

Contributors

Jan V. R. Belcher, PhD, RN
Associate Professor
Wright State University
College of Nursing
Dayton, OH

Suzanne Hetzel Campbell, PhD, APRN, IBCLC
Assistant Professor
Fairfield University
School of Nursing
Fairfield, CT

Wonshik Chee, PhD
Assistant Professor
University of Texas at San Antonio
College of Engineering, Department of Mechanical Engineering
San Antonio, TX

John M. Clochesy, PhD, RN, FAAN, FCCM
Independence Foundation
Professor of Nursing Education
Case Western Reserve University
Frances Payne Bolton School of Nursing
Cleveland, OH

Patricia Fedorka, PhD, RN
Assistant Professor
Duquesne University
School of Nursing
Pittsburgh, PA

Kimberly S. Glassman, MA, RN
Director of Care Management
New York University Medical Center
New York, NY

Linda M. Goodfellow, PhD, RN
Assistant Professor
Duquesne University
School of Nursing
Pittsburgh, PA

Julie Heringhausen
BSN Student
University of Michigan
School of Nursing
Ann Arbor, MI

Carol Holdcraft, DNS, RN
Assistant Dean
Wright State University
College of Nursing and Health
Dayton, OH

Bette K. Idemoto, MSN, RN, CCRN, CS
Clinical Nurse Specialist
University Hospitals of Cleveland
Cleveland, OH

Eun-Ok Im, PhD, MPH, RN, CNS
Associate Professor
University of Texas at Austin
School of Nursing
Austin, TX

Trudy Johnson, MA, RN, CNAA
Vice President, Innovation
   Strategies
New York Presbyterian Hospital
New York, NY

Judith A. Lewis, PhD, RNC, FAAN
Virginia Commonwealth University
School of Nursing
Richmond, VA

Mary L. McHugh, PhD, RN
Associate Professor & Director,
   Professional Development
University of Colorado Health
   Sciences Center
School of Nursing
Denver, CO

Mary Etta C. Mills, RN, ScD, CNAA, FAAN
Director, Professional and
   Distributive Studies
University of Maryland
School of Nursing
Baltimore, MD

Cindy L. Munro, PhD, RN
Associate Professor
Virginia Commonwealth University
School of Nursing
Richmond, VA

Eun-Shim Nahm, PhD, RN
Assistant Professor
University of Maryland
School of Nursing
Baltimore, MD

Carol M. Patton, DrPH, RN, FNP
Assistant Professor & Coordinator,
   FNP Program
Duquesne University
School of Nursing
Pittsburgh, PA

Natalie Pavlovich, PhD, RN
Professor
Duquesne University
School of Nursing
Pittsburgh, PA

Barbara M. Resnick, RN, PhD, CRNP, FAAN
Associate Professor
University of Maryland
School of Nursing
Baltimore, MD

Laree J. Schoolmeesters MSN, RN
Nurse Educator
Pittsburgh Mercy Health System
School of Nursing
Pittsburgh, PA
and Doctoral Candidate
Case Western Reserve University
Frances Payne Bolton School of
   Nursing
Cleveland, OH

Diane J. Skiba, PhD, FAAN
Associate Professor & Health Care
  Informatics Option Coordinator
Project Director,
  The I-Collaboratory:
  Partnerships in Learning
University of Colorado Health
  Sciences Center
School of Nursing
Denver, CO

Nola Stair, MBA
Instructional Design Technologist
University of Maryland
School of Nursing
Baltimore, MD

Meredith Wallace, PhD, APRN
Assistant Professor
Fairfield University
School of Nursing
Fairfield, CT

Carolyn F. Waltz, PhD, RN, FAAN
Professor and Associate Dean for
  Academic Affairs
University of Maryland
School of Nursing
Baltimore, MD

Introduction

Joyce J. Fitzpatrick

Nurse educators, clinicians and scientists are rapidly adapting teaching, practice and research to the many resources available on the Internet. This book is designed as a resource for all nurses who want to use the Internet more effectively in their work as researchers.

For ease of use, the book is divided into 3 parts. Part I includes attention to accessing information online. Part II includes information about conducting research online. Part III informs the reader about how to teach research courses online. Each of these parts includes substantial content that will assist the new and experienced researcher and clinician to make the best use of the internet for scientific and teaching purposes.

Part I includes content that goes beyond beginning access to Internet resources, as much of this information can be found through usual Internet searches. Rather, Part I includes chapters that orient the reader to the more sophisticated methods of accessing information through the Internet. Key resources that are described include the clinical access to online data that will influence evidence-based practice and electronic access to theses and dissertations. Also, the researcher is helped to develop information literacy and to improve techniques for database searching.

Part II prepares the researcher for conducting research online. Techniques for subject recruitment and for data collection via the Internet are presented. Research collaboration is a hallmark of success in clinical research and the Internet presents unique opportunities for advancing such collaboration.

Further, Part II contains many specifics useful to both the novice and experienced Internet researcher. Readers will gather information about how to conduct surveys using the Internet, and will have access to information about the common pitfalls of conducting research through the Internet. One of the key chapters includes information to advise researchers about the Institutional Review Board issues that may be raised with Internet-based research, and another highlights key funding sources for research on the Internet. Issues such as hardware and software options and security in Internet research add depth to the discussion and present content that is essential for the researcher to understand.

Part III is focused on the teaching of nursing research via the Internet, including teaching at the undergraduate, master's, and doctoral level as well as the use of the Internet for teaching research in a continuing education format. Since the teaching of research is only as good as the research application in practice, there is additional attention in this section to research utilization models and their application in both nursing education and clinical practice.

Several appendices complement the core content of the text. Appendix 1 includes samples of Internet-based research projects of several types: survey research, intervention research, and qualitative research. Appendix 2 includes the web resources to enhance nursing research including sources of nursing theory, electronic textbooks, and writing resources.

Throughout the chapters nurse researchers and students of research will find helpful information so that they can maximize the resources available to them through the Internet. The topics included, while not exhaustive, address the questions and issues most frequently raised in relation to Internet use for research.

Part I

Accessing Information Online

Chapter 1

Developing Information Literacy

Kimberly S. Glassman

T he Internet, accessible through the World Wide Web, e-mail, and other communication links, continues to expand our world by providing vast amounts of information from a variety of sources. The Internet has linked researchers and educators for a number of years, and now the possibilities for using the Internet for research are limitless. Researchers have used the Internet to connect to electronic libraries on university campuses, and now are using the Internet as a methodology for sample selection, data collection, and analysis (Adler & Zarchin, 2002; Lakeman, 1997; Thomas, Stamler, Lafreniere, & Dumala, 2000; Yeaworth, 2001). Electronic publishing has become an alternative to traditional print publications. E-mail, chat rooms, listservs and discussion groups all offer researchers advantages not available in the past. All of these utilities provide nurses with opportunities to gain information efficiently and to use new technologies to explore research methods of the future.

USING THE INTERNET TO OBTAIN RESEARCH INFORMATION

An initial step in obtaining research information through the Internet is to conduct a literature search. The basic process of searching begins with selecting a topic or question to research. The user must then divide the topic or question into concepts, find key words or phrases that are relevant to the topic of interest, and then enter them into the search tool.

A starting point for nurse researchers and students is to use an electronic bibliographic database, such as CINAHL or MEDLINE to search the professional literature. The Cumulative Index to Nursing and Allied Health Literature (CINAHL) began in the 1950s, although the electronic version covers the period from 1982 to the present. This database includes all aspects of nursing, allied health, alternative medicine, and community medicine. The MEDLINE database is produced and maintained by the National Library of Medicine, and contains more than 10 million records. Nurses may also find databases such as PSYCHInfo, from the American Psychological Association, ERIC, from the Educational Resources Information Center, and Sociological Abstracts, from the American Sociological Association, to be useful databases for studies in these areas. In addition, EMBASE contains over 3,500 Elsevier Science journals, and is useful for biomedical and pharmaceutical publications. Health and Psychosocial Instruments and UMI's dissertation abstracts are other tools that help finalize a comprehensive literature search, and ensure that adequate studies are being retrieved in a topic area. University and health science center libraries typically have subscriptions to these databases, through services such as *Ovid*, which provides access to full-text journals. Several articles and Web sites are available which describe these databases in more detail (Haynes, 1997; Morrisey & DeBourgh, 2001).

Health sciences librarians are considered to be the experts in guiding nurse researchers and nursing students through the maze of electronic materials available. Most academic health sciences center libraries, as well as public libraries, offer workshops for patrons to learn search skills. There are Web sites that provide tutorials to nurses on how to conduct a literature search on the Internet using specific topic examples (http://library.med.nyu.edu/library/libinfo/classes/nursing.html) and more extensive explanation of various search tools (Sparks & Rizzolo, 1998). Because each electronic bibliographic database has its own search methodology, a consult with a medical librarian ensures that potentially important studies are less likely to be missed.

Keeping abreast of research topic information is time-consuming, yet can be handled efficiently with Internet tools. Subscriptions to free Internet services such as the *Morbidity and Mortality Weekly Reports,* Medscape's Medpulse, and various discussion lists or listservs from professional nursing and specialty groups are ways to receive e-mailed information on a personal computer on a regular basis (Bischoff & Kelley, 1999). Discussion groups can provide an electronic communication link to nurse researchers with shared interests (see Nursing Discussion Forums at http://www.ualberta.ca/%7Ejnorris/nursinglists/). NurseRes, hosted by Kent State University, is a listserv for nurses with an interest in research. For qualitative researchers, Qual Page (http:// www.qualitativeresearch.uga.edu/ QualPage) provides useful information, an opportunity to query other researchers, and links to publications for qualitative health researchers. Those listservs that offer a "digest" version that provides all of the daily messages in one e-mail, limit the volume of e-mail received. McCartney (1999) provides some strategies for nurses wishing to join a listserv, including discussion list "netiquette," maintaining confidentiality, and posing questions to the discussion group. Other Web sites, such as those for statistical analysis software and bibliographic reference management, provide useful information on their Web sites, including software assistance and electronic updates.

Through an affiliation with universities and health facilities, students and faculty can obtain free subscriptions to journal services, such as Ingenta, that e-mail the table of contents from a variety of professional nursing journals or search the literature for recently published articles based on a variety of user-defined search terms (http://www.ingenta.com). This is particularly useful for faculty and graduate students who wish to have weekly or monthly updates of literature searches on user-defined search terms and tables of contents from journals. The "My Library" feature of many academic libraries also offers links to a user's frequently-read full-text journals, as well as updates of new journals and texts available through the library (Wilson, 2001).

The Internet provides a global perspective to researchers interested in sharing research topic information with colleagues in other parts of the world. The immediate nature of global communications can occur in real time, in the form of chat rooms and instant messaging. Listservs are a common method for researchers with common interests to post queries and share information. The qualitative analysis software company, QSR International, provides a listserv for users of NUD*IST and later generation software (Richards & Richards, 2000). This listserv functions as a truly global community, where online assistance and advice is discussed among users from several countries, including the United States, Canada, Australia, Britain, and various European countries. An obstacle to this perception of global community, however, is the use of English as the language for communication, thus limiting this community to those who are English-speaking.

STRENGTHS/WEAKNESSES OF USING THE INTERNET TO SUPPORT RESEARCH

The strengths of using the Internet to support research are 1) access to vast amounts of information and 2) efficiency in obtaining that information. The explosion of Web-based information provides ready access to volumes of primary sources and studies. This strength, however, also serves as a major weakness, in that reviewing the sites/articles retrieved is often more time-consuming than users can manage. The "bookmark" or "favorites" feature of many browsers can serve to facilitate immediate access to preferred Web sites, particularly government or professional society Web sites that update their content on a regular basis. Sites that provide information for time-limited research funding are best searched regularly using this quick-link feature. E-mail services that alert users to new information on a topic, or auto-search features in database collections services, such as Ovid, are ways to receive a continual stream of the latest information in a topic area.

Major weakness of using the Internet for research are the impression that the Internet provides an exhaustive supply of information and nurses' lack of expertise in information literacy (Estabrooks, O'Leary, Ricker, & Humphrey, 2003; Rosenfeld, Salazar-Riera, & Vieira, 2002). University librarians are quick to remind students and faculty that full-text articles are often only indexed in electronic databases beginning in the mid-nineties, and that the indexing of electronic citations is not always comprehensive. Searching multiple databases is imperative, in addition to using less common databases, such as those from other disciplines. Most electronic library databases common to nurse researchers include CINAHL and MEDLINE. However, limiting a search to these popular sites eliminates journals from other disciplines that are often essential to nurses researching topics such as psychosocial adjustment or medical errors. Nurse historians, nurse theorists, and doctoral students are but a few researchers best served by a combination of print media catalogued in libraries, interlibrary loan, and document delivery services, in addition to electronic sources.

Information literacy describes an ability to use appropriate technological tools to obtain information, and includes the ability to critically appraise that information (Rosenfeld et al., 2002). The explosion of Internet-based tools, on the Web or through libraries and commercial sources, adds to the confusion as to where information is best obtained. Nurse researchers and students who limit themselves to popular sources such as MEDLINE and CINAHL will miss important information from government sources such as CRISP and National Institute of Nursing Research (Sparks, 1999). The National Institutes of Health (NIH) database, the Computer Retrieval of Information on Scientific Projects (CRISP), provides detailed information on research grants funded by NIH (Bair, Brown, Pugh, Borucki, & Spatz, 1996).

There are several considerations to using the Internet to support nursing research. The availability of appropriate equipment and the costs of equipment maintenance must be considered. Having the latest equipment and software makes managing information more efficient. Universities now require students to have their own computers, and most academic settings have numerous computer labs to provide additional access for students and faculty.

SUMMARY

The Internet offers a rich opportunity for nurses to gain knowledge and information to support research efforts. Internet access is available in universities, hospitals and clinics, public areas, such as restaurants and transportation centers, and in many homes. The challenge for nurse researchers and students is no longer accessibility, but rather how to sift through reams of material to efficiently find the best data to support the research topic. Internet tools such as electronic library databases, full-text journals, professional societies and government Web sites, funder's Web sites, listservs, and discussion groups can all help students and researchers manage vast amounts of information that can be used to support their research.

REFERENCES

Adler, C. L., & Zarchin, Y. R. (2002). The "virtual focus group": Using the Internet to reach pregnant women on home bed rest. *JOGNN—Journal of Obstetric, Gynecologic, & Neonatal Nursing, 31,* 418–427.

Bair, A. H., Brown, L. P., Pugh, L. C., Borucki, L. C., & Spatz, D. L. (1996). Taking a bite out of CRISP strategies on using and conducting searches in the Computer Retrieval of Information on Scientific Projects database. *Computers in Nursing, 14,* 218–226.

Bischoff, W. R., & Kelley, S. J. (1999). 21st century house call: The Internet and the World Wide Web. *Holistic Nursing Practice, 13,* 42–50.

Estabrooks, C. A., O'Leary, K. A., Ricker, K. L., & Humphrey, C. K. (2003). The Internet and access to evidence: How are nurses positioned? *Journal of Advanced Nursing, 42,* 73–81.

Haynes, C. C. (1997). Nursing & the Net: Exploring world wide opportunities. *AWHONN Lifelines, 1,* 28–33.

Lakeman, R. (1997). Using the Internet for data collection in nursing research. *Computers in Nursing, 15,* 269–275.

McCartney, P. R. (1999). Internet communication and discussion lists for perinatal nurses. *Journal of Perinatal & Neonatal Nursing, 12,* 26–40.

Morrisey, L. J., & DeBourgh, G. A. (2001). Finding evidence: Refining literature searching skills for the advanced practice nurse. *AACN Clinical Issues, 12,* 560–577.

Richards, T., & Richards, L. (2000). QSR N5 (Version 5). Victoria, Australia: QSR International.

Rosenfeld, P., Salazar-Riera, N., & Vieira, D. (2002). Piloting an information literacy program for staff nurses. *CIN: Computers, Informatics, & Nursing, 20,* 236–241.

Sparks, S. M. (1999). Electronic publishing and nursing research. *Nursing Research, 48,* 50–54.

Sparks, S. M., & Rizzolo, M. A. (1998). World Wide Web search tools. *Image: The Journal of Nursing Scholarship, 30,* 167–171.

Thomas, B., Stamler, L. L., Lafreniere, K., & Dumala, R. (2000). The Internet: An effective tool for nursing research with women. *Computers in Nursing, 18,* 13–18.

Wilson, M. D. (2001). Flying first class or economy: Classification of electronic titles in ARL libraries. *Portal: Libraries and the Academy, 1,* 225–240.

Yeaworth, R. C. (2001). Use of the Internet in survey research. *Journal of Professional Nursing, 17,* 187–193.

Chapter 2

Techniques to Improve Database Searching

Laree J. Schoolmeesters

D evising a search strategy for a nursing research topic involves assessment of the topical area, planning the search strategy, performing the search, and evaluating the outcomes or search results. A literature search is cyclic, thus, it is often necessary to modify the search. This chapter provides tips for each phase of the search strategy, identifies major healthcare databases such as Cumulative Index to Nursing and Allied Health Literature (CINAHL) and PubMed, and identifies a variety of online journals, tutorials, and fact sheets.

ASSESSMENT OF THE RESEARCH TOPIC

Free Text Vocabulary

The researcher begins by assessing the topic and its depth and scope. Formulate a topic statement. For example: "What has been published about nursing research and the use of the computer?" This will lead to a list of topic words or phrases. When using a search database, these may be referred to as subject headings, keywords, or free-text (Schloman, 2000). Be descriptive with words and phrases, using a thesaurus or a colleague's insight. In the above example, keywords may include "nursing research" or "nurse research" and "computer" or "technology."

Controlled Vocabulary

Another method to consider is using controlled vocabulary, which is used on many health databases such as CINAHL and PubMed. Controlled vocabulary is a hierarchical system of subject headings developed by the database. In PubMed this is called the Medical Subject Heading (MeSH). The MeSH tree structure has 16 broad headings arranged alphabetically and hierarchically, e.g., anatomy, diseases, and health care. The headings become increasingly more specific (Medical Subject Headings, 2002). About 70% of CINAHL headings also appear in PubMed (Ovid, 2003b).

To use controlled vocabulary, go to the MeSH Browser home page at http://www.nlm.nih.gov/mesh/MBrowser.html and enter a topic of interest. The search can be limited to main headings, qualifiers, Supplementary Concept Records (chemical thesaurus), or all of the above. The Search MeSH Annotations/Scope Notes automatically come with any search that used the button "all of the above." One can ignore the limits underneath "Search in these fields of chemicals," unless of course that is the topical focus (Medical Subject Headings, 2002).

The search will produce a MeSH descriptor data sheet that displays the MeSH heading, tree number, annotation (information similar to the topic heading, but may not be pertinent to the search), scope note (a brief definition of the word), entry terms (which may contain the original word searched, along with other similar terms), allowable qualifiers (e.g., adverse effects [AE], economics [EC]), and a unique ID. Anything that is highlighted can be clicked to provide additional information. The descriptor data sheet will not automatically link to PubMed or another database, though the findings will enhance a search on the PubMed system. The MeSH terminology and fact sheet can be downloaded from the home page at this Web site (Medical Subject Headings, 2002).

PLANNING THE SEARCH

The planning phase includes making decisions about the kind of information to retrieve. The most common resources are journals and textbooks, but can include dictionaries, government documents, and dissertations. These resources may be online or in print form. The plan should also include an overall discipline focus such as nursing, medicine, or psychology. These decisions will locate the most pertinent database, though searching among multiple databases may be needed with very narrowly focused topics or to get different perspectives from various domains (Schloman, 2000). In planning, examine the following health databases and online journals to find the most appropriate avenue for a specific search.

Health Databases

There are a number of health databases to select and search. The following is a sample of available databases: PsycINFO, CANCERLIT, CINAHL, and PubMed/MEDLINE. Most of these require a subscription fee except PubMed/MEDLINE, which is free, subsidized by taxpayers. A brief description will be given of PsycINFO, and CANCERLIT, with a more in-depth look at CINAHL, and U. S. Government Healthcare Databases, which includes PubMed/MEDLINE.

PsycINFO and CANCERLIT

PsycINFO is a compilation of all psychology related information, which includes, for example, medical, nursing, and education disciplines. This database dates back to 1872 and is updated weekly (Ovid, 2002). CANCERLIT has all pertinent information on cancer and was developed by the U. S. National Cancer Institute. This database began in 1975 and continues to the present. A large number of these records have abstracts and many records can be found on MEDLINE (Ovid, 2003).

CINAHL Database

CINAHL is an online searchable index of primarily nursing information. Journals from allied health fields include: cardiopulmonary technology, physical and radiologic technology, surgical and occupational therapies, social and emergency service, medical and laboratory, medical assistant, medical records, and physician assistant. Publications include 1200 journals, many with abstracts, and 7000 full text articles. There are 29 print journals available online. Almost 100 research instruments with 23 full text instruments are also available (Levy, 2002). Additional types of publications are books, software, dissertations, conference proceedings, standards of practice, and audio-visual materials. The database began in 1982 and is updated monthly (Ovid, 2003). Access is by fee and usually a workplace or a college library holds a subscription; if not one can access the CINAHL support Web site at http://www.cinahl.com to purchase a subscription (Thede, 2003).

CINAHL Web site. The cinahl.com Web site, though not the searchable database, has several areas of interest, such as CINAHL sources, the library, and CINAHL direct, which can enhance a CINAHL search. The site offers a free demonstration of a search with registration. It also offers an online user manual and other helpful tools (CINAHL information systems, 2003).

CINAHL sources. This area offers Web sites related to topics on allied health, alternative therapies, biomedical, case management, consumer health, critical care, evidenced-based medicine, health administration, health informatics, library resources, medical equipment and supplies, mental health, nursing, and pharmacology. After clicking on a topic, selections of Web sites are identified, each with a clickable link and a description of the organization and the Web site, such as the authors of the site, the audience, and general content (CINAHL information systems, 2003).

The library. Click on Journal List to get an alphabetical listing of all CINAHL journal holdings or click on Journal Directory to view journals by discipline or field (e.g., women's health), by categories or subsets (e.g., peer reviewed), by country of publication, or by subject (e.g., nursing, research). Click on Document Types to locate publications being indexed. These generally include journals, books, audiovisual, pamphlets, software, dissertations, or research instruments. Another feature is descriptions of topical subheadings, which may be searched in full or with two letter codes. Generally the codes match MeSH subheadings (CINAHL information systems, 2003).

CINAHL Searching Tips

In the CINAHL database, click on "Subject Heading" to determine where the topic word places in the hierarchy. This displays more general and specific terms that help identify other avenues or keywords of a search. This feature also notes how many citations are found, which determines if a search needs to be exploded or focused. By checking either box, the next step in the search results in subheading possibilities, such as education, contraindications, or evaluation, which can help refine the search. If the search produces a vast number of matches, use the limit functions. The limits include latest update, research abstracts, English, full text, revised date, PDF, images, CE Module information, and setting time limits on the publication date (Ovid, 2003).

To search for one of the almost 100 research instruments, type in the topic and click search, then type in "limit 1 to research instrument." The number "1" refers to the first topic search. This limiting works for legal cases, journal articles, and accreditation (Levy, 2002).

U. S. Government Databases

MEDLINE/PubMed Database. MEDLINE/PubMed is the U. S. National Library of Medicine's (NLM) bibliographic database and encompasses the fields of medicine, nursing, dentistry, veterinary medicine, the health care system, and the preclinical sciences. MEDLINE contains references and abstracts from 4,600 biomedical journals published in 70 countries and the U. S., most in English. The database contains over 12 million citations from the mid-1960s to the present, including about 130,000 population-related entries. PubMed has links to full text articles. Over 50% of the records have abstracts (MEDLINE, 2002c; Ovid, 2003c).

PubMed Central. PubMed Central (PMC) is the NLM's literature archive for health care professionals life of the sciences journal. PMC contains journals only. Research-based journals are required to be peer-reviewed (PubMed Central, 2003).

PubMed Searching Tips

"The NLM Gateway allows a search in multiple retrieval systems at the U.S. National Library of Medicine (NLM). Retrieval systems include: MEDLINE/PubMed, OLDMEDLINE, LOCATORplus, MEDLINEplus, ClinicalTrials.gov, DIRLINE, Directory of health organizations, Meeting Abstracts, and HSRProj." (NLM Gateway, 2001, p. 1). Typing in a key term and clicking "go" will provide search results divided into types of material, such as journals; books, serials, and AV materials; consumer health; meeting abstracts; and other collections. It is extremely important to set limits (field searching) when using PubMed as it contains a vast number of records. Setting limits includes types of material, English only, dates of publication, and subsets (AIDS, bioethics, history of medicine, and space life sciences). Some convenient features are found in the displayed search. First, it links relevant articles. Second, articles can be ordered online. Third, citations can be e-mailed (NLM Gateway, 2001).

Combined Health Information Databases. The Combined Health Information Databases (CHID) is a searchable Web site produced by the National Institutes of Health (NIH), Centers for Disease Control and Prevention (CDC), and Health Resources and Services Administration (HRSA). This database contains 16 topics on health information and health education resources. It is updated four times a year (CHID Online, 2003).

ClinicalTrials.gov. This site provides an online search for clinical research studies. It includes privately and government funded research in humans. The site provides information on the trial's purpose, sample, geographic location, and telephone numbers for more specific information (ClinicalTrials.gov, 2003).

LocatorPlus. This site is an online catalog for books, audiovisuals, and journal titles available through the NLM. It has a straightforward simple search and an easy-to-use advanced search. The site also has an online tutorial (LocatorPlus, 2003).

Online Healthcare Journals

Online healthcare journals are an easy way to obtain information quickly. At Linkout (2003), there is a list of journals with links to full-text Web sites. Linkout is part of the NLM system. Journals are listed alphabetically or by title. Some are fee based or may require a user registration.

The University of Iowa has compiled a list of healthcare journals that offer free online articles. Some are print journals that are also placed online. Most rely on the PubMed database. There is a helpful search button, but the search system is actually quite forthright. Clicking on the selected journal links to the PubMed directory or the CINAHL online journal directory (Hardin MD, 2002).

IMPLEMENTING THE SEARCH

Boolean Logic

Boolean, searching is a simple method of using words, also called terms or operators, such as "AND," "OR," and "NOT," to combine the selected topic keywords within the search boxes on the internet database (Cooper, 2000; Elkordy, 2002). The Boolean operators will broaden or narrow the search. Boolean terms may be used in basic searches, although some search engines require use of the advanced mode. If an initial keyword alone search retrieves only a few hits (lingo for information that matches the topic), broaden the search using Boolean terms "OR" and "AND" "OR" is best used for two similar keywords that describe the topic, for example beginners "OR" students. "AND" will find articles that contain both words, for example nursing "AND" research. To narrow or make a search more specific use exclusion terms such as "NOT," for example nursing "NOT" nurses (Cooper, 2000). The following symbols can sometimes be used interchangeably, for example, "+" for "AND" or "−" for "NOT" (Elkordy, 2002).

Proximity Operators

Proximity operators, phrasing, or use of parentheses can also be helpful to pinpoint a topic. Proximity operators "NEAR" or "ADJ" help keep topic search words close together. For example "nursing" and "research" may appear in the same text of a journal though paragraphs apart. To use a proximity operator, type ADJ/2 in addition to the topic words. This lets the search engine know that the topic words must be within two words of each other (Elkordy, 2002). To use phrasing, the topic words are put in quotes, for example "nursing research," which keeps them together. The use of parentheses (called nesting) in a search is a similar method to keep words together (Cooper, 2000; Elkordy, 2002).

Truncation, Wildcards, and Stemming

The ultimate goal of using truncation, wildcards, and stemming is to find all forms of the search word. Truncation uses the shortest form of the word such as nurse, which would also find nurses, nursing, and nursed (Cooper, 2000). Some search tools use plurals, though not all. To ensure the search includes both singular and plural topic words, use a wildcard or stemming (a typed symbol) such as an asterisk (*) or an ampersand (&). This technique allows any ending for the word, for example "research*" would look for researches, researching, researched, etc. Not all search tools will allow this technique, however (Elkordy, 2002).

Field Searching

"Databases are collections of records organized in a similar manner; simply put, this means they are divided into fields that contain the same information in each record" (Elkordy, 2002, p. 5). Field-specific searching is crucial to find appropriate matches. Most databases contain check boxes or pull-down menus that will define the fields, for example: published within the last 5 years, specific journals or authors, or articles in English only.

EVALUATING AND MODIFYING THE SEARCH RESULTS

Search Troubleshooting

If the search is not returning matches, one can consider some of the following problems. One of the most common is misspelling or typographical errors. If the search is producing unusual subject areas the topic may need to be reconceptualized or one can try using the help function in the database. Also, be cognizant that a meta-search engine may strip the Boolean terms or field operators. If the search results are overwhelming, narrow the topic, for example try "mid-range nursing research" instead of "nursing research." If the search results are nonexistent try eliminating extraneous material or make topic words more general. For example, try "nursing research theory" instead of "Florence Nightingale nursing research grand theory" (Elkordy, 2002).

Tutorials

The Internet offers a vast amount of easily accessible knowledge, especially in the arena of healthcare databases. Using Boolean logic and limit searching will enhance and refine any search. Using tutorials can improve search results. Both CINAHL and PubMed have tutorials that can be accessed online. The CINAHL direct user's manual has a multitude of practical information on basic and advanced searches. It has sample images of how to use CINAHL. This information may be printed (CINAHL information systems, 2003). For continued improvement in search skills examine the following tutorials that were located in Elkordy (2002) and Cohen's (2003) Web sites:

1. Flanagan, D. (2003). Finding it online. At: http://home.sprintmail. com/~debflanagan/main.html contains search skills, information on how to use various search engines, and a scavenger hunt to apply newly acquired knowledge.
2. Cohen, L. (2003). *Internet tutorials.* At: http://library.albany.edu/ internet/sponsored by the University at Albany libraries. The site has 20 tutorials on various aspects of research and use of the Internet.
3. Cooper, C. (2000). *The Internet & IT for busy nurses & therapists.* At: http://www.carol-cooper.co.uk/book/chapter02.shtml.
4. Dwyer, C. (1997). *Pointers for making the most of your Medline searches.* At: http://www.acponline.org/journals/news/oct97/ medline.htm Assists in using MeSH terms for a research topic.
5. Elkordy, A. (2002). *Web searching, sleuthing and sifting.* At: http:// www.thelearningsite.net/cyberlibrarian/searching/lesson1.html. Offers 6 lessons in Internet searching with assignments.
6. *Finding information on the Internet: A tutorial teaching library Internet* workshops sponsored by Teaching Libraries of University of California, Berkeley. At: http://www.lib.berkeley.edu/ TeachingLib/Guides/Internet/FindInfo.html.
7. Leita, C. (2003). *Search tools chart & search engines quick guide* At: http://www.infopeople.org/search/chart.html. Developed by the Infopeople Project, supported by the U.S. Institute of Museum and Library Services. This is a 2-page table containing information on search engines, metasearch engines and subject directories along with corresponding database sizes, Boolean and other search options, and miscellaneous special features.
8. Schloman, B. F. (2000). *Searching the nursing literature.* At: http://class.kent.edu/public/kent365/index.html. Designed for Kent State University Students, but guests are provided with a login ID and password free of charge.
9. Sullivan, D. (Ed.). *Search engine math.* At: http:// searchenginewatch. com/facts/math.html. Maximize searches using basic tips. Also click on Web searching tips.
10. *The Spider's Apprentice: How to Use Web Search Engines,* by Monash Associates. At: http:// www.monash. com/spidap.html. Ranks search engines for ease of use.

11. Thede, L. Q. (2003). *Informatics and nursing: Opportunities & challenges* 2nded.). At:http://junior.apk.net/lqthede/Informatics/ Chap17/Chap17.htm.

REFERENCES

CHID Online. (2003). [Web site] Retrieved July 3, 2003, from http://chid.nih. gov/index.html

CINAHL information systems. (2003). [Web site] Retrieved July 3, 2003, from http://www.cinahl.com/

ClinicalTrials.gov. (2003). [Web site] Retrieved July 3, 2003, from ClinicalTrials.gov.

Cooper, C. (2000). *The Internet & IT for busy nurses & therapists.* Retrieved July 3, 2003, from http://www.carol-cooper.co.uk/book/chapter02.shtml

Cohen, L. (2003). *Internet tutorials.* Retrieved July 3, 2003, from http://library. albany.edu/internet/ Updated: June 2003

Elkordy, A. (2002). *Web searching, sleuthing and sifting.* Retrieved July 3, 2003, from http://www.thelearningsite.net/ cyberlibrarian/searching/lesson1.html.

Hardin, M.D. (2002). *Free medical journals: PubMed search.* Retrieved July 3, 2003, from http://www.lib.uiowa.edu/hardin/md/ej.html

Levy, J. R. (2002). Searching the CINAHL data base part 2: Abstracts, cited references, and full text. *CINAHLnews, 21*(2), 11. Retrieved July 3, 2003, from http://www.cinahl.com/library/library.htm

Linkout. (2003, July). Retrieved July 3, 2003, from http:// www.ncbi.nlm.nih.gov/ entrez/journals/loftext_noprov.html

LocatorPlus. (2003, June, 23). Retrieved July 3, 2003, from http://locatorplus.gov/

Medical Subject Headings. (2002, March 5). [Web site]. National Library of Medicine. Retrieved July 3, 2003, from http://www.nlm.nih.gov/mesh/ meshhome.html

MEDLINE. (2002, March 22, 2002). [Web site]. *National Library of Medicine.* Retrieved July 3, 2003, from http://www.nlm.nih.gov/databases/databases_ medline.html

NLM Gateway. (2001, May 24). Retrieved July 3, 2003, from http://gateway.nlm. nih.gov/gw/Cmd

Ovid. (2002). *Ovid Technologies Field Guide on PsycINFO.*

Ovid. (2003a). *Ovid Technologies Field Guide on CancerLIT.*

Ovid. (2003b). *Ovid Technologies Field Guide on CINAHL.*

Ovid. (2003c). *Ovid Technologies Field Guide on MEDLINE.*

PubMed Central. (2003). [Web site]. *National Library of Medicine.* Retrieved July 9, 2003, from http://www.pubmedcentral.nih.gov/

Schloman, B. F. (2000). *Searching the nursing literature.* Retrieved July 3, 2003, from http://class.kent.edu/public/kent365/index.html

Thede, L. Q. (2003). *Informatics and nursing: Opportunities & challenges* (2nd ed.). Retrieved July 3, 2003, from http://junior.apk.net/~lqthede/formatics/ Chap17/ Chap17.htm

Chapter 3

Evidence-Based Practice: Getting Online Information in the Clinical Setting

Trudy Johnson

The ten rules for the 21st century healthcare system defined in a 2001 Institute of Medicine (IOM) report included the principles that decision-making is evidence-based, safety is a system property, and knowledge is shared and information flows freely (IOM, 2001). Pursuit of clinical inquiry and utilization of research will foster the future of quality and patient safety in healthcare by applying these principles. Managing complex patient care requires clinicians to integrate in their practice clinical experience, knowledge, reasoning, and judgment. The application of the research process and research findings in nursing practice enables nurses of all experiential levels to achieve optimal care outcomes and strive for clinical excellence.

Clinicians must constantly rethink and redesign traditional care delivery to meet the challenges of new diagnostic, technological, and treatment modalities for patient care. Evidence-based practice supports clinicians and administrators in making important decisions for changing care delivery. Employing evidence-based practice is one of five core competencies for healthcare professionals to meet the challenges of the current practice environment. This requires the integration of the best research with clinical expertise, patient values and participation in learning and research activities to the extent possible (Greiner & Knebel, 2003).

EVIDENCE-BASED PRACTICE

Evidence-based practice is a systematic process for finding, evaluating, and applying contemporaneous research findings in clinical problem solving and decisions. The basic steps include formulating a clear question based on a clinical problem, searching the literature for the best available evidence, evaluating the strength of that evidence, and implementing useful findings in clinical practice based on valid evidence (Rosenberg & Donald, 1999). The value of evidence-based nursing practice assumes that optimal nursing care is provided when nurses, the interdisciplinary team, and other decision-makers have access to the latest research and a consensus of expert opinion, with consideration of cultural and personal values. This approach to nursing care allows clinicians to bridge the gap between the best evidence available and the most appropriate nursing care of individuals, groups, and populations with varied needs (Sigma Theta Tau International, 2003).

Currently the Internet is a useful facilitator of the transfer of knowledge and information. The Internet allows researchers to disseminate knowledge rapidly and expansively around the world, while enabling the clinical inquiry for the application of research findings in practice. Whatever an individual's clinical specialty or interest there are numerous means for ensuring practice is current with the latest research. Furthermore, for clinicians who are seeking to improve quality and patient safety, the Internet offers opportunities to interact with other healthcare professionals they would not have access to on a day-to-day basis.

SKILLS FOR RESEARCH UTILIZATION AND EVIDENCE-BASED PRACTICE

According to Benner's Novice to Expert Model, research utilization and evidence-based nursing occur differently based on the experience of the nurse (Benner, Hooper-Kyriakidis, & Stannard, 1999). For novice nurses who are students or recently employed as practicing nurses, use of research will augment learning as they gain experience in organizing their work, developing essential skills, and applying knowledge. As the novice becomes increasingly competent, they have an augmented understanding of clinical situations that allows them to recognize the clinical relevance of changes in signs and symptoms to a greater degree than before.

For the competent nurse to become proficient, utilization of research and evidence-based nursing will enhance the transition to a clinical grasp of pattern recognition and skilled know-how for managing critical interventions. The expert nurse is more intuitive in his or her practice-based response to clinical reasoning, anticipating change, identifying problems, problem solving, and engaging appropriately with patient or family (Benner, et al., 1999). Thus, based on knowledge and experience, the ability to seek and apply research appropriately varies from nurse to nurse.

Competent nurses can validate the appropriateness of their day-to-day practice by reviewing current research findings available on the Internet. One can subscribe to online journals or review multiple journals for subjects of interest and then purchase individual articles. This allows the nurse to ensure their practice is consistent with findings in the literature. Publications of significant research findings are important to review from the original source. Because there are few regulations regarding posting information on the Internet, one should always access the original source and not rely on information that is summarized in lay newspapers or that is interpreted by another researcher. As a nurse's practice evolves, it should include expanding the search of research findings to literature reviews and sharing those findings with colleagues in an interdisciplinary forum to solve problems and seek improvements to care.

Expert or advanced practice nurses are ideal to provide leadership in the clinical setting in the conduct and utilization of research. Competency and computer proficiency should be encouraged among all healthcare clinicians. When proficiency is obtained, clinicians can be encouraged to use the Internet in everyday practice and to implement clinical change based on evidence. The integration of literature reviews or the use of meta-analyses can provide the foundation for conducting scholarly research or recommending clinical redesign of care protocols or processes.

METHODS OF INFORMATION EXCHANGE

Expert knowledge sharing includes both reactive and proactive processes. One can react to information one may hear from other sources such as the news media, journals, Internet listservs, or personal e-mail that present information regarding new research findings. Individuals may then search for that information on the Internet. Information may be immediately accessible on the Internet or require a financial transaction to obtain either a download or a hard copy in the mail. Another reactive process results from the desire to acquire clinical knowledge on a subject or to improve clinical practice based on evidence, which requires systematic literature review that is done through the virtual medical and nursing libraries available online.

Receiving information on an ongoing basis requires proactively participating in listservs and receiving e-mails from various journals that have relevant subjects of interest for the user. Clinicians affiliated with an organization that is a member of a healthcare consortium such as Premier, Voluntary Hospitals of America (VHA), or University Health-System Consortium (UHC) may access the consortium proprietary Web sites that provide online access to databases of information as well as listservs for different subjects. Professional organizations also have listservs that enable the participant to receive information targeted for their specific area of interest based on the population that the professional organization is associated with (e.g. American Pain Society, Oncology Nurses Society). Participating in listservs frequently provides information about research and a network that may span the world consisting of professionals who are willing to discuss the merits of evidence currently under review.

The use of online journals is essential as an individual proactively receives information about research or reactively seeks information. Every clinician should identify journals that are most valuable in their clinical practice and review these journals regularly. Electronic notices of abstracts of new research via e-mail are sometimes available without a journal subscription for current abstracts in upcoming publications. The clinician can either seek the article in a library or purchase a copy via the Internet if the individual or associated employer does not currently subscribe. For individuals who are affiliated with an academic facility one may be able to access full-text journal articles from a work or educational organization. An excellent example of this was during the Severe Acute Respiratory Syndrome (SARS) outbreak in 2003 when the *New England Journal of Medicine* published a free full -text article on the current findings about the epidemiology and treatment of SARS from a panel of experts. Subscribers to the journal's e-mail alert system received this article on the day of publication. Clinicians were able to use this information to develop internal guidelines for hospitals located in high-risk communities. Communication with other professionals via e-mail and listservs provides rapid discussions across the country or internationally in a manner that would have taken months 15 years ago. The interaction and exchange of ideas with other healthcare and nursing professionals can lead to further inquiry and evidence to support change.

FINDING THE EVIDENCE

To conduct evidence-based practice there must be sufficient research published on a specific topic. Nurses must then apply the necessary skills in accessing and analyzing the available research and then be able to implement changes based on the evaluation of the evidence. It is beyond the scope of this chapter to discuss the implementation of research findings, but the critical factor is the skills to find adequate resources that address a specific topic and how to access that information to perform an appropriate analysis. The clinician who wants to increase his or her knowledge for personal growth and development, find treatment options for a patient, or conduct a literature review to formulate a research question, can easily use the Internet to conduct this type of inquiry with the requisite skills.

The ability to use search engines effectively is essential for finding primary and secondary reports of research. General search engines such as Google or Yahoo can provide information about non-profit organizations (e.g. American Cancer Society), medical societies (e.g. American Academy of Allergy, Asthma, and Immunology), nursing societies (e.g. Sigma Theta Tau) and government agencies (e.g. Department of Health and Human Services) that provide links to research findings and information on clinical trials. However, the most effective search engines for healthcare research are targeted search engines such as the National Library of Medicine's PubMed.

Internet search engines are designed with advanced search functions using Boolean logic that is common to library databases. Boolean searching is based on a system of symbolic logic developed by George Boole, a 19th century English mathematician. Performing a Boolean search requires one to enter keywords that best describe the topic to yield an accurate search with fewer irrelevant documents. Information is available on the Internet regarding Boolean logic and individuals can also use a tutorial/online help function. Otherwise, one may seek a professional librarian for advice on how to optimize the use of these databases.

An alternative to search engines is familiarity with databases on the Internet such as those found at http://www.Cochrane.org. The Cochrane Library offers Cochrane Reviews which provide in-depth literature reviews by subgroups such as for breast cancer, HIV, or pain. Reviews include summaries of the literature conducted by experts and overseen by a quality assurance panel. Cochrane Reviews do not substitute for individuals evaluating the quality of research findings, but instead enable them to refine their own searches more rapidly. To supplement these reviews, other Web sites provide additional sources of broad-scoped information and some specialty Web sites provide information of a more narrow focus.

Web sites that have a broad scope of information include government sponsored sites such as the Agency for Healthcare Research and Quality (AHRQ) (http://www.ahrq.org) or the National Institute of Nursing Research (NINR) (http://www.nih.gov/ninr/). AHRQ sponsors evidence-based practice centers that support the development of clinical practice guidelines based on evidence and include Web links to academic centers sponsored by AHRQ with information for a variety of clinical specialties.

When an adequate body of research has been obtained the Internet can be used for further analyses or discussion among e-mail groups or listservs. The National Guideline Clearinghouse™ (NGC™) NGC-L electronic discussion list is one example. This forum provides healthcare professionals and others an opportunity to discuss issues related to clinical practice guideline development, methodology, research, dissemination, implementation, and use of guidelines (http://www.guideline.gov/resources/discussion_list.aspx.).

Increasingly guidelines are being integrated in clinical decision support tools based on clinical evidence developed from a consensus evaluation by a panel of experts. The Internet offers an alternative to the knowledgeable user in healthcare organizations that do not have clinical information systems with software for decision support or access to other knowledge-based proprietary software. Organizational Intranets frequently include access to Web sites that are reliable sources of guidelines for clinical practice and other sources of evidence for clinical decision-making such as the aforementioned Web sites from government agencies or professional societies. By providing hyperlinks, institutional Intranets facilitate access and assist the user in finding reliable information for evidence-based practice.

VALUE OF INTERNET USE IN CLINICAL PRACTICE

The value of the Internet is self-evident in providing access at the point of care. Additional advantages include easier access to information when compared to books and journals, particularly when a traditional library is not readily available; the scope of searching is broad and draws from many databases simultaneously; and new research is immediately available as it is published. Disadvantages include a limited number of journals in full text format, the need for broadband connectivity to conduct rapid searches, and the necessary journal familiarity the user must have to specific sources of information and patient populations. Overall, the benefits have enabled clinicians to support evidence-based practice more readily across all clinical settings from community-based to academic healthcare settings.

REFERENCES

Benner, P., Hooper-Kyriakidis, P., & Stannard, D. (1999). *Clinical wisdom and interventions in critical care.* Philadelphia: W. B. Saunders.

Institute of Medicine. (2001). *Crossing the quality chasm.* Washington, DC: National Academy Press.

Greiner, A., & Knebel, E. (Eds.). (2003). *Health professions education: A bridge to quality.* Washington, DC: National Academy Press.

Rosenberg, W., & Donald, A. (1995). Evidence-based medicine: An approach to clinical problem solving. *British Medical Journal, 310,* 1122–1126.

Sigma Theta Tau International Position Statement on Evidence-based Nursing; Retrieved June 2003, from http://www.nursingsociety.org.

Chapter 4

Electronic Theses and Dissertations

Linda M. Goodfellow

I nnovations in technology afford graduate students the opportunity to prepare and submit their thesis or dissertation in electronic format. Similar to the traditional, print-and-bound copy, electronic theses and dissertations (ETDs) are created using a standard word processor. When the final version is completed and approved, the thesis or dissertation is converted to portable document format (PDF) and submitted electronically to a Web page on the library's server where it is stored. The ETD offers graduate students a new way of presenting their work and a new way for the academic community to view a student's work. There is a growing trend among universities to pursue ETD projects.

HISTORICAL BACKGROUND

In 1997, Virginia Polytechnic Institute and State University, commonly known as Virginia Tech, was the first university to require its graduate students to submit the thesis or dissertation as an electronic document (Eaton, Fox, & McMillan, 2000). Since then, several universities have also adopted the same policy. Other universities have made it an option whereby students can choose to submit their work electronically or in the traditional printed version. Accessed through a university's computer network system, the Networked Digital Library of Theses and Dissertations (NDLTD), or UMI ProQuest Digital Dissertations (Moxley, 2001), ETDs offer significant benefits to graduate students and both new and seasoned scholars.

Conceptualized in 1987, the NDLTD was developed to support theses and dissertations in an electronic format (Moxley, 2001). Housed at Virginia Tech, the NDLTD was the first digital library created to provide worldwide, free, instantaneous access to graduate students' research. The NDLTD initiative emerged as a result of a collaborative effort of universities and the support of government agencies, private companies, and other organizations (Suleman, Atkins, Goncalves, France, & Fox, 2001). Since 1996, over one hundred universities (United States and international universities), institutions, regional centers, and organizations have joined the NDLTD initiative. There is no cost to join. Its global appeal is evident from the number of countries in Africa, Asia, Central and South America, and Europe that are represented. In addition, over 8,500 ETDs are available via the NDLTD (Suleman et al.). Over 2,800 of these have been submitted by Virginia Tech's graduate students (Eaton et al., 2000). Most of these can be found through a federated search engine that was developed by a group of graduate students in computer science, also from Virginia Tech (Bolander, 2001).

UMI ProQuest Digital Dissertations offers institutional subscribers online access to those dissertations published since 1997 (UMI ProQuest Digital Dissertations, 1999). UMI, formerly known as University Microfilm Inc., has been the central repository and disseminator for North American printed theses and dissertations for the past 50 years. Since 1997, all printed versions of theses and dissertations received are scanned and converted to electronic versions by UMI so that they can be accessed through their database. UMI also offers access to Dissertation Abstracts, a database that includes more than 1.6 million entries (UMI ProQuest Digital Dissertations).

ADVANTAGES AND CONCERNS RELATED TO ETDS

The benefits and opportunities that ETDs offer will become evident to the nurse over the next few pages as the traditional bound thesis or dissertation is compared to the electronic version. As with any new idea or change in tradition, there are also concerns and obstacles to overcome. These too will be addressed.

ETDs benefit the academic community and provide opportunities to graduate students that were once unfathomable. As more and more universities require graduate students to submit their research electronically and become members of the NDLTD, these benefits and opportunities will be further realized. According to Fox (1999), ETDs have changed the future of academia.

Unfortunately, traditional bound theses and dissertations are rarely read by anyone other than the graduate student's faculty advisor and committee members (Young, 1998). Unless the graduate student publishes his or her research in a scholarly journal, results of the study may never be shared with the academic community. If the research is published, it may take one or even two years after the student graduates before it actually appears in print. In some disciplines, by the time it's read, the research is outdated.

Immediate access to the graduate student's work is one of the many advantages of ETDs. Thus, new ideas and meaningful results generated through graduate research work are readily available for electronic review much sooner than are the printed versions. ETDs also have the potential to reach a much wider audience in a timelier manner than do printed versions (Eaton et al., 2000). Graduate students, faculty researchers, nurse educators, hospital administrators, and nurses in clinical practice can all benefit from ETDs. ETDs are quickly becoming a valued resource to nursing scholars interested in the most up-to-date research by graduate students.

Universities and their individual schools also benefit from the broad and immediate exposure ETDs can offer. University name recognition, the quality of the research produced, and the prestige that often accompanies research will be an invaluable recruiting tool for both graduate students and new faculty members. Schools of nursing, for example, can showcase state-of-the-art research by creating a link from their Web page to the graduate student's ETD.

ETDs also provide students the opportunity to learn valuable computer skills and, through online submission, gain experience in electronic publishing (Moxley, 2001). Students can enhance their presentations as well as their communication skills with the multimedia capabilities ETDs have to offer. Opportunities for creative expression (Young, 1998), not possible with printed versions, are endless for those students who submit their work electronically.

Most ETDs still look similar to the printed version. They include the usual preliminary pages, five or more chapters, figures, tables, references, appendixes, and one-inch margins. This will change. The inclusion of hypertext links, interactive elements, and multimedia elements will eventually become common. Linked Excel tables and inserted visuals will provide simple ways to create richer, more appealing theses and dissertations (Moxley, 2001). Many graduate students are already taking advantage of the multimedia capabilities offered by ETDs. For example, a graduate from Virginia Tech included 42 sound clips of parrot calls in her dissertation (Young, 1998).

Consider some of the conceptual and complex issues that are explored in nursing. Also, think about how difficult it can be to thoroughly explain a concept or describe the efficacy of an intervention in words without losing the beauty of discovery. One can only imagine the scenarios and visual images that could further define or illustrate the research findings if the ETD also included sound and colorful interactions.

Critics of ETDs are not convinced that all graduate students have the ability to communicate electronically and think that to require ETDs is unfair (Young, 1998). Others are concerned that the computer skills of some faculty are not up to par. However, creating an electronic document from a basic word processing file is not difficult and neither is the online submission process. Universities offer ETD workshops, create online manuals, and include specific instructions on their library servers.

Critics also argue that a graduate student's research is not ready for electronic publication until it undergoes the rigor associated with peer review (Fox, 1999; Young, 1998). Others are concerned that ETDs may hinder future publication of the student's research in scholarly journals (Fox & McMillan, 1997). Justifiably so, publishers often frown upon prior publication. Although it is conceivable that an editor could reject an article because of prior publication on the Web, distribution as a dissertation is very different from publication in a refereed journal (Moxley, 2001). In addition, converting a dissertation into a publishable manuscript requires extensive work. Although the substance of the dissertation must be maintained, the writing style and format may differ because of editorial preferences, extraneous information must be eliminated, and the length of the manuscript may be cut by one hundred or more pages. By the time the manuscript is completed it generally does not look or even read like the original thesis or dissertation (Fox & McMillan, 1997).

In 1997, criticism from both scholars and graduate students led administrators at Virginia Tech to modify their ETD requirement (Young, 1998). Although still required to submit their thesis or dissertation electronically, students were given options whereby they could choose one of three levels of access: 1) submit the entire work for immediate worldwide access; 2) submit the entire work for access only by authorized users of the university; and, 3) submit the entire work but prevent its access for a period of time (Young, 1998). Other universities requiring ETDs have also adopted the same or similar options for students.

At Duquesne University, students are permitted to delay worldwide or university access for one year for copyright or patent purposes. This provides students with an adequate amount of time to publish their research in a scholarly journal or apply for a patent, common in disciplines other than nursing such as physics or chemistry. Students are encouraged to consult with potential editors prior to deciding which level of access is best for them.

Saving precious shelf space in university libraries is another advantage of ETDs. By saving shelf space and thus, avoiding binding costs, libraries will also save money (Bolander, 2001). Some students do not see this as an advantage because they would like to have their bound thesis or dissertation included with the hundreds of others. Although tradition is nice, shelf space in any library is limited and very few theses or dissertations are ever removed from the shelf for reading. In addition, unless the interested scholar has access to the library where the bound copy is shelved, printed theses and dissertations are often difficult to obtain (Young, 1998). One can request an interlibrary loan from the library of the university where the student graduated, or order a copy from UMI. Unfortunately this may take several days or weeks (Mizzy, 2001). Failure to locate a bound copy is also a real possibility.

An ETD, on the other hand, can be quickly accessed at no cost from the university's library via their Web page and the NDLTD if the University from which the student graduated is a member. Electronic dissertations can also be ordered from UMI ProQuest Digital Dissertations, although a small fee is attached (Teper & Kraemer, 2002).

Long-term retention of ETDs has also raised concerns. Whereas a printed version may collect dust, it is durable and stable over time. Should anything ever happen to the original, UMI through microfilming can provide universities with a backup of the printed version (Teper & Kraemer, 2002). ETDs differ from traditional theses and dissertations in that there is no paper or microfilm backup. Electronic documents also differ from paper because access and delivery will change with time. In addition, electronic archiving has not yet been established and decisions are being made without specific guidelines (Teper & Kraemer).

Most universities require students to create a CD-ROM of their electronic work and submit it to the universities library as a backup. But, as computer technology and software change, will the CD-ROM be a reliable method of backup? If not, and other procedures are not in place, it may be that valuable research is lost forever. Ultimately it will be the responsibility of universities requiring ETDs to provide the resources necessary to preserve electronic versions of theses and dissertations (Teper & Kraemer, 2002).

The ETD can also benefit the student after graduation. Easy access makes the ETD a valuable marketing tool. Students can link the ETD to their resume via the web address of their university's library or the NDLTD. Potential employers benefit by having the opportunity to evaluate the candidate's research interests and writing skills prior to offering an interview or a position. Digital libraries also provide headhunters, private companies, universities, and institutions a mechanism by which to search for potential employees. Tenure and promotion committees would also value a frequently accessed and cited thesis or dissertation (Moxley, 2001).

GUIDELINES FOR ETD SUBMISSION

The general procedures associated with the ETD submission are similar from one university to another. Most use the same basic guidelines originally set forth by Virginia Tech (http://etd.vt.edu) and the NDLTD (http://www.ndltd.org). The interested nurse is encouraged to visit these Web sites, as well as Web sites from other universities requiring ETDs such as Duquesne University (http://www.library.duq.edu/etd), University of California, Berkeley (http://www.library.berkeley.edu/), or West Virginia University (http://www.library.wvu.edu/etd). A wealth of information can be obtained directly from these Web sites with links to other resources if additional information is needed.

Once the graduate student has defended their research and obtained final approval from their chairperson and committee members, the ETD submission process can begin. The following describes the process used to submit an ETD and provides answers to frequently asked questions related to ETDs. This information was obtained from the ETD Collection, Duquesne University, Gumberg Library Electronic Theses and Dissertations Web site at http://etd/library.duq.edu/ETD-db/help/ (2002).

Converting a Document to Portable Document Format (PDF)

Created with word processing software, the thesis or dissertation must be first converted to Portable Document Format (PDF). This format is necessary to ensure that the ETD looks the same when viewed by different Web browsers and operating systems. For instance, if the file were not converted to PDF then fonts, pagination, tables, graphs, etc. would not necessarily appear to others like the original paper version. In addition, the ETD must be in PDF for inclusion on the library servers and the NDLTD.

In order to open and then read a PDF document, Acrobat Reader must be installed on a computer. This application is free from Adobe and can be downloaded from http://www.adobe.com. To convert a document to PDF, the Adobe Distiller can be used. This is available in the same package as Adobe PDFWriter, which is different from the Acrobat Reader. The Adobe PDFWriter can be downloaded from the Adobe homepage after a fee is paid. Documents created in Microsoft Word can be converted to PDF(http://www.etd.uc.edu/content/pdf/Word2PDF.pdf.

There are several additional ways to convert word-processed files to PDF as well. A program called Ghostscript can be downloaded to your computer free of charge from http://graduate.gradsch.uga.edu/etd2/ghost.htm. Although a physical printer is not necessary to use Ghostscript, a PostScript printer driver will need to be installed on your computer. A free generic printer driver can be downloaded from Adobe at http://www.adobe.com/support/downloads/main.html.

A file can also be converted to PDF on the Web without downloading any additional software at http://docmorph.nlm.nih.gov/docmorph. This requires an Internet connection during the conversion process. Depending on the size of the file, it may take a considerable amount of time to convert, especially if a standard dialup connection is being used.

Creating an Account

Once the thesis or dissertation has been converted to PDF, students submit the ETD via a Web page on the library's server of their university. Students must first create an account on the login page by choosing a username and password. Once an account is created the same username and password can be used to make any changes that may be necessary for the library to approve the ETD. This also permits the student to complete the submission process over a period of time rather than at one sitting. An ETD status message will keep the student on track throughout the submission process. This message will let the student know what they have already done and what still needs to be completed prior to library approval.

The security system used by most universities requires the student's browser to support cookies. A cookie is information about a user or session that is stored in a cookies.txt file by a compatible browser. In this case, a cookie stores the student's username and password. Once logged in, a cookie allows the student to move from page to page in the ETD process without the need to log in repeatedly. Most browsers come with cookies enabled. If for some reason cookies are not enabled or were disenabled for one reason or another, instructions that accompany the browser will provide the directions to enable cookies.

Adding Files

A Web browser is required to upload files during the ETD submission process. All versions of Netscape greater than 3.0 and all versions of Internet Explorer greater than 4.0 will support file uploads. A correct file name must be used and should not contain any spaces or slashes. If the student is submitting more than one file, the files will be sorted alphanumerically on the title page that will present the student's information on the Web. Thus, to guarantee that the files appear in a specific order, it is important to name them accordingly with two digit numeral codes in front of them. For example: 01titlepage.pdf, 02acknowledgements.pdf, 03introduction.pdf, and so forth.

If the browser is using a proxy server of any kind, file uploads will not work properly. A proxy is used to permit access between networks. Proxy settings can be changed for most browsers and directions to do so can be found by consulting the browser's help files. Some versions of America Online (AOL) use this type of proxy to connect to the Internet. If the student uses AOL, they will need to download a newer version of either Netscape or Internet Explorer to their computer and use it along with their AOL account. Additional information can be obtained at http://www.lib.vt.edu/extended/extendedcamp.html#dbs.

Entering Keywords and Abstract

At some point in the ETD submission process, students will be directed to enter keywords or phrases that describe their thesis or dissertation in the appropriate field in the browser window. It is important to select keywords that are not already in the abstract or title page. Those words will already be indexed for searching. By providing different search terms, access to the ETD will be improved.

The abstract can be entered directly into the abstract field in the browser window or the student can copy and paste the abstract from a standard word processing program. If the copy and paste method is preferred, then the equivalent HTML entity must be used because special characters such as & (ampersand), < (less than), or > (greater than) will not be displayed correctly in a browser window. HTML entities will however display special characters correctly. An HTML entity consists of an ampersand (&), a word or number, and a semicolon (;). For example, the HTML equivalent to & is "&," < is "<," and > is ">." A complete list of HTML entities is maintained by the World Wide Web Consortium and can be viewed at http://www.w3org/ MarkUP/HML3/latin1.HTML

Access Options for ETDs

As part of the ETD process, students are asked to complete a form online that will indicate their preference in regard to others accessing their thesis or dissertation. This form may vary depending on the university's ETD requirements. Generally, however, students can choose to make the full text available with unlimited access, available for their university only, or unlimited access after a set period of time, usually one year. Students can also limit access to specific sections, an entire chapter, or even a diagram for a set period of time, if they wish.

SEARCHING FOR ETDS

ETDs are available through universities' databases and online catalogs. They are also available through the NDLTD library (http://www.theses.org) and UMI ProQuest Digital Dissertation database (http:// wwwlib.umi.com/cre-search/gateway/mail/).

Bound Copies

Most graduate students will usually want to have a bound print copy of their thesis or dissertation. Also, bound copies are often given to committee members or others who may have played a significant role in the dissertation process. These can be still ordered through UMI ProQuest in much the same way as the traditional printed versions were ordered before ETDs existed. Students can also print the number of copies they want bound and have a local print shop do the binding.

Copyright Requirements for ETDs

Copyright requirements for ETDs are no different than those for the traditional print version of the thesis or dissertation. Permission must be
obtained to use copyrighted material regardless of the version used.
Copyrighted material must also be cited according to copyright holder's
requirements (Crews, 2000).

Since an ETD is an expression of the student's original work, it can
be copyrighted. This holds true even if some of the text has already
appeared in journals or books and copyright to the publisher was
relinquished for previously published material. The parts copyrighted by
others, however, must be properly cited according to the publisher's
requirements (Crews, 2000). Additional information on copyright and fair
use can be obtained at several Web sites including the Copyright Clearance Center (http://www.copyright.com), Copyright Law and Graduate
Research (http://www.umi.com:8090/hp/Support/DExplorer/copyright),
and the United States Copyright Office Library of Congress
(http://lcweb.loc.gov/copyright).

Completing the ETD Process

Library staff are vital in the ETD submission process. Most universities
have guidelines that appoint one or several of the library staff responsible for checking the student's files for completeness and accuracy. If
something is left blank or incorrect, they will notify the student by e-mail.
Once the ETD has been converted to PDF and uploaded to the library's
server, the library staff will further verify that the file is readable. If for
some reason it is not, the student will be notified and asked to resubmit
the PDF file. Most university libraries have established key personnel to
troubleshoot any problems that may arise. They are available to answer
questions, offer suggestions, and make the ETD process as easy as
possible for the student.

The Role of Education in ETDs

Like many new and innovative ideas, change takes time and is often accompanied with some degree of angst and skepticism. One of the biggest
obstacles faced by universities that are committed to the ETD process is
getting students and faculty to buy into it. Universities who require ETDs
have the responsibility for educating students and faculty alike by offering

workshops, in-services, online training courses, and hands-on experience (Fox, 1999). Students and faculty must also take responsibility for their own learning by attending the classes offered, reading some of the articles written about ETDs, visiting the ETD Web pages on university library servers, and navigating the digital libraries available.

Through education ETDs will eventually become second nature. This chapter was written to provide nurses, whether they are graduate students, members of the academic community, or clinicians, with a better understanding of ETDs. As more schools of nursing require their graduate students to submit ETDs, digital databases including ones found in university libraries, the NDLTD, and ProQuest Digital Dissertations will become invaluable Internet resources for nurses.

REFERENCES

Bolander, R. C. (2001). Virginia Tech improves access, saves money and shelf space with electronic theses and dissertations. *OCLC Newsletter*, 22–25.

Crews, K. D. (2000). *New media, new rights, and your new dissertation.* ProQuest Information and Learning Copyright Law & Graduate Research. Retrieved May 20, 2003, from http://www.umi.com:8090/ hp/Support/ Dexplorer/copyright/ Part1.html

Eaton, J., Fox, E., & McMillan, G. (2000). Results of a survey of Virginia Tech graduates whose digital theses and dissertations are accessible worldwide. *Council of Graduate Schools Communicator, 33*(9). Retrieved January 7, 2002, from http://www.cgs.org

ETD Collection. (2002). Retrieved May 20, 2003, from Duquesne University, Gumberg Library Electronic Theses and Dissertations Web site: http://etd/library.duq.edu/ETD-db/help/

Fox, E. (1999). Networked digital library of theses and dissertations. *Nature Web Matters, 12.* Retrieved July 3, 2003, from http://www.nature.com/nature/ webmatters/library/library.html

Fox, E. A., & McMillan, G. (1997). Request for widespread access to electronic theses and dissertations. *NDLTD.* Retrieved January 11, 2003, from http:// www.ndltd.org/info/request.htm

Mizzy, D. (2001). ETD: Bringing dissertations (and theses) to your desktop. *The University Library System Digital Library News, 12.* Retrieved January 7, 2002, from http://www.library.pitt.edu/about/newsletter/issue12/

Moxley, J. M. (2001). Universities should require electronic theses and dissertations. *Educause Quarterly, 3,* 61–63.

Suleman, H., Atkins, A., Goncalves, M., France, R., & Fox, E. (2001). Networked digital library of theses and dissertations: Bridging the gaps for global access—

Part 1: Mission and progress. *D-Lib Magazine.* Retrieved July 3, 2003, from http://www.dlib.org/dlib/september01/suleman/09suleman-pt1.html

Teper, T. H., & Kraemer, B. (2002). Long-term retention of electronic theses and dissertations. *College & Research Libraries, 5,* 61–72.

UMI ProQuest Digital Dissertations. (1999). About ProQuest Digital Dissertations. *Digital Dissertations.* Retrieved October 22, 2001, from http://wwwlib.umi.com/dissertations/about_pqdd

Young, J. R. (1998). Requiring theses in digital form: The first year at Virginia Tech. *Chronicle of Higher Education.* Retrieved July 11, 2003, from http://chronicle.com/data/articles.dir/art-44.dir/issue-23.dir/23a02901.htm

Part **II**

Conducting Research Online

Chapter 5

An Overview of Research Methods Using the Internet

Kristen S. Montgomery

The Internet has been increasingly used as a research methodology. Many methodologies exist that are appropriate for use via the Internet and still maintain integrity of a research project. It is likely that research methodologies using the Internet will continue to grow and expand in coming years and that new research methodologies will be developed and tested. This chapter provides a brief overview of the most prevalent Internet-Based research methods. Subsequent chapters provide more detail on some of these methods.

Survey research is by far the most common methodology used in Internet-based research. However, intervention studies are becoming more commonplace as the science, technology, and expertise of the researchers continue to advance. Qualitative methodologies are being used as well. The literature includes reports of both in-depth descriptive qualitative interviews and virtual focus groups.

SURVEY RESEARCH

Internet-based surveys can be conducted online with interactive surveys that can be completed and submitted directly to the researcher or with survey forms that are downloaded and then mailed, faxed, or e-mailed by attachment to the researcher. One-to-one interviews between the researcher (or research assistant) and the participant may also take place via e-mail or in chat rooms (Eysenbach & Wyatt, 2002). A survey may also be sent by attachment to e-mail groups. Surveys that are mailed back to the researcher can generally be anonymous with only the city and state of postmark apparent. Faxes have less security in that generally a fax number appears on the received fax, which can then be traced to the phone line from which it originated. This can lead to an individual's home or place of business. Even when a service is used to send the fax (e.g., Kinko's) the respondent's general location or city is revealed. Use of e-mail is even less rigorous than either mail or fax responses. E-mail is much easier to trace and personal information may be gathered from the Internet Service Provider (ISP). Thus, if one plans to use the Internet to conduct survey research, they need to be aware of these issues. However, it is a viable methodology that may be used with Internet-based research.

Interestingly, Gueguen and Jacob (2002) found that participants in their Internet-based survey responded more readily to complete a survey when the identification of the person requesting the survey was considered to be of high status (e.g., a scientist) when compared to someone of lower status (e.g., an undergraduate student). Perhaps participants in this study assumed that something would come of a research project that was being conducted by an individual who was more experienced and was conducting the research as part of their job, whereas an undergraduate student might not be viewed as serious regarding the likelihood that the project would be completed, in which case the participant's time would have not been put to good use. The survey was sent to both students and people at random. The authors did not compare these two groups to any other groups where the credentials of the person requesting the survey were unknown.

Marsden and Jones (2001) discussed the use of procedures to ensure that Web-based questionnaires that will be used online for survey research would be evaluated for reliability and validity. The authors described a comparison study where 16 female participants between the ages of 19–49 completed a Web-based questionnaire and then repeated the questionnaire using a paper version to establish reliability and validity of the two methods. The authors found that all nine of the questionnaires tested were suitably useful to be placed on the Web for use in research.

The Internet may also be useful in increasing the overall response rate by adding an additional data collection site via the Internet. For example, Andersson, Lindvall, Hursti, and Carlbring (2002) conducted a study to explore the presence of a relatively rare condition known as hyperacusis (an unusual intolerance of ordinary environmental sound). The authors surveyed a random group of individuals and obtained a response rate of 59.7% ($n = 589$) via postal mail and 595 individuals who viewed a banner advertisement self-recruited to complete the survey online for a 51.9% response rate. Thus, the authors in this study effectively doubled their sample size by including an Internet-based form of the survey.

White and Hauan (2002) identified that while Web-based data collection has many benefits, the quality of the data collected can sometimes be less than desirable. Because Web-based data collection is essentially unsupervised, the researcher will not have knowledge of any problems or misinterpretations that occur among subjects who complete an online instrument unless there is a mechanism to provide feedback via e-mail or other means. White and Hauan note that using time stamps when subjects complete online surveys can help researchers determine if difficulty was encountered and subjects returned to the questionnaire at a later date/time. Of course, this method is not foolproof, but it does offer some advantage to not using time stamps.

INTERVENTION RESEARCH

Intervention research is considered the gold standard to make changes in practice. After several years of introductory research using the Internet, research projects and topics have progressed to the intervention stage. While this methodology is just beginning to be used in Internet-based research, it is likely to grow in coming years. Internet-based intervention research includes both interventions that are provided online, and studies in which participants are randomized to the intervention group, which includes an Internet component. The intervention can be delivered via the Internet or the intervention can be an education on how to use the Internet (Edgar, Greenberg, & Remmer, 2002).

QUALITATIVE METHODS

In-Depth Descriptive Interviews

While a few papers were identified that described the results of qualitative in-depth descriptive interviews using the Internet (e.g., Clark, 2002; Chou, 2001), no articles were identified that addressed methods in conducting qualitative interviews online via e-mail, chat rooms, or HTML formats. It is likely that because the goal of qualitative research is to examine an experience in-depth, researchers may not wish to rely exclusively on use of the Internet to meet these goals. Additionally, the crucial role of the interviewer/researcher in qualitative research and the mutual interaction between participant and research is difficult to support in studies that might occur online.

Virtual Focus Groups

Virtual focus groups have been described in the literature to obtain in-depth information from participants on a topic of interest and to link similar participants to each other to form social support networks (Adler & Zarchin, 2002). In the study by Adler and Zarchin, the researchers posed a series of sequential focus-group questions to participants over a 4-week period, which is different from a traditional focus-group that is generally covered in one session. Thus, participants were allowed more time for reflection than is common among traditional, in-person focus groups. Using this technique, researchers were able to gather rich and detailed qualitative data (Adler & Zarchin). However, data generated from traditional focus groups may need to be differentiated from virtual focus groups, given the differences in response times and the fact that participants may not be interacting with each other or the researcher directly.

NEW RESEARCH METHODOLOGIES USING THE INTERNET

Eysenbach and Wyatt (2002) wrote about using the Internet as a research methodology by reviewing materials posted on a Web page as a valuable resource to understand people and the social and cultural contexts in which they live. The authors noted that this type of approach allows researchers to examine individuals outside of experimental settings (Eysenbach & Wyatt). Information that is posted by individuals on bulletin boards or in chat rooms may be useful to researchers who want to understand more about health beliefs, common topics of discussion, motivation, and emotional needs. However, care is warranted in collecting "data" when participants are not aware they are involved in a research study.

SUMMARY

As a method of research, the Internet offers several advantages including rapid access to potential participants, access to difficult-to-reach populations, openness among respondents, and potentially reduced research costs (Rhodes, Bowie, & Hergenrather, 2003; Eaton & Struthers, 2002). Participant privacy, particularly when sensitive data is being collected, and convenience are additional potential benefits of using the Internet as a research methodology (Baer, Saroiu, & Koutsky, 2002; Eaton & Struthers, 2002). Challenges to use of the Internet as a research methodology include the fact that not all potential participants have access to or use the Internet, competition for the respondent's attention by other sites of interest, biased samples, and limitations in the generalizability of results (Rhodes, et al., 2003). As Internet-based research methodologies move into the future, additional research is needed that compares these new and emerging methodologies to previously tested and refined methods (Katz, et al., 2002).

REFERENCES

Adler, C. L., & Zarchin, Y. R. (2002). The "virtual focus group": Using the Internet to reach pregnant women on home bed rest. *Journal of Obstetric, Gynecologic, and Neonatal Nursing, 31,* 418–427.

Andersson, G., Lindvall, N., Hursti, T., & Carlbring, P. (2002). Hypersensitivity to sound (hyperacusis): A prevalence study conducted via the Internet and post. *International Journal of Audiology, 41,* 545–554.

Baer, A., Saroiu, S., & Koutsky, L. A. (2002). Obtaining sensitive data through the Web: An example of design and methods. *Epidemiology, 13,* 640–645.

Chou, C. (2001). Internet heavy use and addiction among Taiwanese college students: An online interview study. *Cyberpsychology and Behavior, 4,* 573–585.

Clark, D. J. (2002). Older adults living through and with their computers. *Computers and Informatics in Nursing, 20,* 117–124.

Eaton, J., & Struthers, C. W. (2002). Using the Internet for organizational research: A study of cynicism in the workplace. *Cyberpsychology and Behavior, 5,* 305–313.

Edgar, L., Greenberg, A., & Remmer, J. (2002). Providing Internet lessons to oncology patients and family members: A shared project. *Psychooncology, 11,* 439–446.

Eysenbach, G., & Wyatt, J. (2002). Using the Internet for surveys and health research. *Journal of Medical Internet Research, 4*(2), E13-E18.

Gueguen, N., & Jacob, C. (2002). Solicitation by e-mail and solicitor's status: A field study of social influence of the Web. *Cyberpsychology and Behavior, 5,* 377–383.

Katz, D. G., Dutcher, G. A., Toigo, T. A., Bates, R., Temple, F., & Cadden, C. G. (2002). The AIDS Clinical Trials Information Service (ACTIS): A decade of providing clinical trials information. *Public Health Reports, 17,* 123–130.

Marsden, J., & Jones, R. B. (2001). Validation of Web-based questionnaires regarding osteoporosis prevention in young British women. *Health Bulletin, 59,* 254–262.

Rhodes, S. D., Bowie, D. A., & Hergenrather, K. C. (2003). Collecting behavioural data using the World Wide Web: Considerations for researchers. *Journal of Epidemiology and Community Health, 57,* 68–73.

White, T. M., & Hauan, M. J. (2002). Using client-side event logging and path tracing to assess and improve the quality of Web-based surveys. *Proceedings of the American Medical Informatics Association,* (AMIA), New York, 894–898.

Chapter 6

Online Subject Recruitment

Suzanne Hetzel Campbell

O pportunities to use the Internet as an adjunct to the research process are continuing to increase and nurse researchers are well positioned to use the Internet as a recruitment method for research projects. The purpose of this chapter is to provide an overview of the advantages and disadvantages of recruiting subjects for traditional research projects via the Internet. Comparisons are made between online recruitment and other types of recruitment.

ADVANTAGES OF ONLINE SUBJECT RECRUITMENT FOR TRADITIONAL RESEARCH PROJECTS

There are many advantages to online subject recruitment; one specifically important for nurse researchers is access to specific, sometimes difficult-to-find populations. Populations that are difficult to recruit related to the sensitivity of the topic may be accessible through the Internet. Additionally, theoretically, the potential for a large and diverse sample exists. A large sample size reduces the risk of Type II errors and increases the potential power of the research (Krantz & Dalal, 2000). Opportunities for data collection are immeasurable. The speed of access to participants is a benefit, with most individuals replying in 2–3 days compared to 4–6 weeks with mail surveys and 2–3 weeks for telephone surveys (Farmer, 1998). When subjects are recruited via the Internet, reminders may be sent for study completion. Participant convenience may also be considered a benefit of online subject recruitment. However, even though recruitment times are enhanced, an individual must still complete the traditional research project. Follow-up or delay in completing the project can sometimes be problematic.

The inclusion of explanatory material in a subject recruitment Web page to explain the purposes of the study, what participation entails, and any compensation that is provided, can prompt respondents to participate in the study. If flexibility is possible in the timing of study completion, that too can be considered a benefit to the participant, which may increase the overall study response rate.

CHALLENGES OF ONLINE SUBJECT RECRUITMENT FOR TRADITIONAL RESEARCH PROJECTS

The nature of the sample that can be recruited via the Internet can be one potential challenge. The Graphic, Visualization, and Usability Center's 10th World Wide Web (WWW) User Survey (Kehoe, Pitkow, Sutton, Agarwal, & Rogers, 1999) indicated the following information about WWW users: they are white (87.2%), male (66.4%), married (47.6%), an average of 37.6 years old, 88% have some college with 59% having at least one degree, and 37% have used the Web for 5 years and access it daily from home (78.7%) or work (68.5%). Thus, online participant recruitment may miss lower socioeconomic and otherwise marginalized groups and potentially result in a nonrepresentative sample.

Although these statistics point to a difficulty in accessing globally representative samples from the Internet, and inherent problems of nonprobabilistic sampling and self-selection exist, the Web, as a recruitment tool, is still in its infancy. Increases in the numbers of female participants, and the wider age distribution of Web samples, demonstrate an increase in external validity and movement toward a more representative group (Krantz & Dalal, 2000). Because of the variability that currently exists between users' computer capabilities, access, operating systems, servers, and browsers, recruitment may vary (Harris & Dersch, 1997). Tracking users through more sophisticated means and collecting information about demographics allow greater generalizability to well-studied segments of the overall population.

COMPARISON OF SAMPLES

Previous research to date has revealed conflicting outcomes in terms of samples obtained. Some researchers have had success in recruiting diverse samples, where others have obtained nonrepresentative samples. Certainly more research needs to be done comparing methods of data collection, but the decreased cost and convenience of subject recruitment via the Internet make it worth exploring.

There are two other issues related to recruitment of respondents via the Internet. One is a sampling issue described by Buchanan and Smith (1999) as "true volunteers." These are individuals who seek out studies to participate in for the intellectual reward. Their motivation and exposure to many studies over time may influence how they respond and ultimately influence study findings. The second issue relates to the perceived anonymity of the respondent who may assume a new identity and provide false demographic and other information. In truth, data falsification can also occur in traditional research methods as well, and cannot be seen as a unique challenge to Internet-recruited samples (Duffy, 2002). In subject online recruitment there are additional methods to protect the anonymity of the subjects. Individuals who volunteer to participate can be given a special identification number or password to access a specific site for data collection. This also can assure that there is only one response per individual.

ONLINE SUBJECT RECRUITMENT

Some basic techniques have been used online to recruit participants for research. Participants may be solicited from newsgroups or lists related to the research topic of interest. For example, researchers interested in recruiting breastfeeding women may go to a lactation support listserv. Those interested in new parents may target parenting sites. Internet communities related to the research topic may have Web sites, e-mail lists, listservs, or electronic bulletin boards where notices about the study can be posted. Identifying sites where the target population is using the Web is key to accessing Internet communities that will provide participants for the study. Providing information on the purpose of the study, benefits and risks to participants, and the researcher's credentials and qualifications can increase the likelihood of individuals participating.

Another technique is to post to search engines or wait for them to find the study with keywords. All Web studies posted will be affected by search engines unless they are protected from general access (Krantz & Dalal, 2000). Identifying groups containing your sample and targeting the gatekeeper(s) to obtain access and to assure your credibility is another technique for recruitment. For many of the groups to be contacted, sensitive topics (sexual behavior), specialized groups (HIV positive individuals), and traumatic experiences (childbirth with poor outcomes) may create difficulty in recruiting willing participants. In addition, participants who have experienced difficult encounters with the health care system may be distrusting of health care providers.

Advertisements in newspapers, lay journals, or the media (radio or TV) can direct potential participants to a Web site that provides information about the study. This might be considered indirect Web recruiting; however, providing information to participants via a Web page might increase the overall participation rate, as potential subjects are able to learn more about the study in a nonthreatening manner prior to enrollment. Previous researchers have reported better success in recruitment if the link to the study Web page or researcher's e-mail is provided on the radio or television Web site after an interview or report of the study (Krantz & Dalal, 2000). Remembering an esoteric Web link or e-mail address given on the air versus clicking on it on the radio or television Web site can greatly affect the activity on the site. One group of researchers found that classified-type advertisements are costly and do not make a noticeable difference in the sample size of completed surveys (Harris & Dersch, 1997).

The new Health Insurance Portability and Accountability Act regulations, enforced in the United States since April 2003, will have an effect on how health information may be used for research purposes. This may affect some of the recruitment techniques utilized through professional organizations and may require more reliance on other methods to recruit participants. For some researchers, a multiple (or hybrid) approach to recruitment produces better results. When a major group of participants can be identified, the gatekeeper for the group can send a postal letter to all members introducing the research project to establish the researcher's credibility. Including some professional background and contact information may also be helpful. Participation in organization activities, like writing a column in the newsletter, is another way to increase researcher credibility and recruit participants. Depending on distribution of such a newsletter, additional participants may be reached for possible recruitment.

When individuals are recruited online, it is possible that additional individuals will be recruited via the snowball technique. That is, individuals who participate in the study tell a friend or family member about the study and then they participate as well. In general, this is okay; however, it is important to know the strengths and limitations of this recruitment method. For example, significant bias can occur in the sample if multiple participants are recruited from one venue and they have unique characteristics. For example, if the study site was sent to a listserv of individuals abused as children, when these individuals present them- selves to participate in the study onsite, it may be that these unique char- acteristics are discovered or they may not be if they are not the focus of the study. To be sure, it may be worthwhile to include one simple question in the study, "How did you find out about this study?" and thereby identify situations that may affect the research results.

CONCLUSIONS

This chapter has provided information for the nurse researcher consid- ering online subject recruitment. Recognizing the limitations of this type of recruitment is important and seeking ways to report the results that adequately reflect the sample reached, methods to enhance sample representativeness, and generalizations of the research results are important as well. Problems of underrepresentation of minorities, women, and older adults in research need creative solutions. To date, recruit- ment via the Internet has not adequately addressed these discrepan- cies. In the future, as the demographics of Internet users changes, recruit- ing underserved populations via the Internet may become a reality. Nursing can be at the forefront in developing methods to recruit these populations via the Internet.

REFERENCES

Buchanan, T., & Smith, J. (1999). Using the Internet for psychological research: Personality testing on the World Wide Web. *British Journal of Psychology, 90,* 125–144.

Duffy, M. E. (2002). Methodological issues in Web-based research. *Journal of Nursing Scholarship, 34,* 83–88.

Farmer, T. (1998). *Understanding this thing we call Internet research.* Retrieved June 9, 2003, from http://infotekonline.com/irgonline/white-paper-on-internet.htm

Harris, S. M., & Dersch, C. A. (1997). Conducting research on the Internet: Poten- tial, concerns and reflections. *Kappa Omicron Nu Forum: Technology, 11*(1). Retrieved June 9, 2003, from http://www.kon.org/forum/harris.html

Kehoe, C., Pitkow, J., Sutton, K., Aggarwal, G., & Rogers, J. (1999). *Graphics Visualization Usability Center tenth WWW user survey.* Retrieved June 9, 2003, from http://www.cc.gatech.edu/gvu/user_surveys/survey-1997–04/

Krantz, J. H., & Dalal, R. (2000). Validity of web-based psychological research. Psychological Experiments on the Internet. In M. H. Birnbaum (Ed.), *Psycho- logical experiments on the Internet* (pp. 35–60). New York: Academic Press.

Chapter 7

Data Collection With Personal Data Assistants

Cindy L. Munro and Judith A. Lewis

P ersonal Data Assistants (PDAs) are among the newest and smallest of devices that can perform many of the same functions as full-sized computers. A major advantage of these small, portable devices is the ability to access and record information at the point of contact with a patient, rather than having to transcribe the information from a stationary computer and transport it to the site of contact in hard copy, make modifications or additional entries on the hard copy, and then enter the revised information back into the stationary computer. The PDA decreases time on tasks, increases efficiency, and prevents transcription error.

USE OF PDAS

Personal Data Assistants are available from a variety of vendors, but most have the same basic functionality. The main differences among devices are operating system (Microsoft Windows CE or the Palm OS), expandability, processor speed, and memory size. Some even come with the ability to record sound files. Lewis and Sommers (2003) described many applications for PDAs including personal organizers, address books, calendar programs, sending and retrieving electronic mail, word processing, spreadsheets, database management, Internet access, and professional presentations. Other more nursing-specific applications discussed by Lewis and Sommers (2003) include medication databases, patient tracking programs, calculators, prescription writing, International Classification of Diseases ICD-9 coding, and accessing textbooks and periodical literature.

While there are differences in functionality among the various types of PDAs, they all perform similar functions. Major differences exist between the two operating systems, Palm OS and Microsoft Windows CE. There are many more medical applications and shareware applications available for those PDAs using the Palm OS, mainly because it has been on the market longer and attracted the attention of third-party software developers earlier. The number of applications for those PDAs using the Windows CE operating system is growing rapidly, and is more likely to have to be purchased for a fee. One advantage to the Windows CE operating system is the availability of Microsoft Word and Excel and the ability to transport files directly from either of those applications between the portable device and a stationary computer.

The ability to create and use spreadsheets and database formats that are compatible with full-version programs, their portability and lack of intrusive appearance, and the ability to record information at the point of contact make them ideal data recording devices for collection and transmission of research data.

USE OF PDAS IN RESEARCH

The use of PDAs as tools to enhance research is relatively new. However, the PDA can be a powerful assistant in a research project. The PDA can be used very effectively in data collection, storage, and management. It can also improve communication among research team members, increase efficiency of scheduling, and provide on-site, easily accessible research study materials. Although PDA use in research has many potential benefits, careful planning and consideration as well as ongoing maintenance and troubleshooting are required.

Data collection activities are an ideal application for the PDA. Data collection forms can be developed in a variety of applications, depending upon study needs and resources. Quantitative data forms may be developed using a variety of PDA programs. One of the most widely used form-generation programs is PenDragon Forms (http://www.pendragonsoftware.com/). PenDragon provides an interface between the PDA and a Microsoft Access database housed on a personal computer. The PDA serves as a conduit of information to the Access database, but PenDragon does not provide for any data analysis to be performed directly on the PDA. Multiple PDAs can be licensed to synchronize with a single Access database, making this program ideal for studies that employ multiple data collectors. A "hot sync" operation immediately stores the collected data onto the PC. This allows immediate access to the data by the researcher. Other forms of data collection, such as an electronic scanning sheet, require a waiting period to have enough forms to score, as well as waiting to have codes deciphered. When the data collector performs a "hot sync" operation, the data is stamped in the database with the PDA identification number and the date and time of the "hot sync." This allows a review of the data for accuracy, missing data, and immediate feedback to individual data collectors. Other spreadsheet programs, such as Microsoft Excel, can be used as data entry spreadsheets with few modifications. Microsoft Excel has basic statistical functions, and many PC-based statistical packages (such as JMP) can import Excel spreadsheets for more sophisticated analysis.

Behavioral or observational data present different data collection challenges. Several programs are available to address this need. Spectator Go! (http://www.biobserve.com/mobile_systems/spectator_go/), BEST, and !Observe are three options. These software packages permit entry of categorical data collected in an observational setting. For example, the investigator developing a data form in Spectator Go specifies behaviors of interest; the time and duration of those behaviors by specific subjects is time-stamped when the behavior is clicked in the PDA. In this case, multiple subjects can be observed simultaneously, and interactive behaviors can be recorded. For example, in Spectator Go, a researcher observing a group of preschoolers could note behaviors of individual children as well as interactions among children all in a single data collection process on a single PDA. However, in this case, the data collection software also does the data analysis, producing summary data, graphs, and tables. While this self-contained analysis is exceptionally user-friendly and may meet the needs of some researchers, it does not permit tailoring of data analysis by the researcher or export of the data to a more powerful statistical package. This limits the ability to do additional or alternative analyses.

Some PDAs have built-in audio recording capabilities. These PDAs can be used to record interviews and transfer these audio files to desktop computers at the time of synchronization.

ADVANTAGES OF PDAS IN RESEARCH

Many programs designed to assist clinicians can also be useful in certain research settings. Clinical tools that calculate specific scores may meet the needs of a particular study. For example, if body mass index (BMI) is a variable of interest, several PDA programs can compute BMI from entered height and weight data. For this type of data calculation, a preprogrammed tool may serve better than a data collection software package. Calculated data can be entered into a PDA data collection form, or entered directly into a PC database.

The standard programs on a PDA may also facilitate the research process, and the ability to update documents with each synchronization of the PDA provides the advantage of all study personnel having complete, accurate, and timely information. Instructions for research personnel, including procedure manuals, can be stored in text documents. Contact numbers can be stored in the memo area. Additional study information, such as personnel responsibilities, study protocols and procedures, and palm tips/troubleshooting instructions can be saved in the memo area or in a text file. This enables all study personnel to have easy and portable access to study documents. A "communication book" can also be created in the memo area to permit study personnel to share information. The memo can be designed to allow only one person (such as the principal investigator or study coordinator) to be able to communicate information or it can be designed to allow multiple users the ability to update or manipulate the memo. A bulleted "to do" list and calendar function enhance tracking of responsibilities assigned and completed.

DISADVANTAGES OF PDAS IN RESEARCH

In considering use of the PDA, investigators are advised to consider several potential issues. First, not all personnel may have familiarity with use of a PDA, and even those who are familiar with the PDA will need study-specific training regarding how the PDA will be used in the specific project. Training of all personnel who will use the PDA includes the basics of use, including procedures for "hot sync," use of the stylus, battery or recharging requirements, password protection, handwriting recognition software, accessing forms and study materials, and troubleshooting. Second, investigators will need to consider whether PDA use will be restricted to study purposes, or whether users will be permitted to keep personal information on the devices as well. Expectations should be clearly communicated to study personnel. If personal PDA use is permitted, clear instructions regarding how to avoid downloading information unrelated to operation of the study into study files is needed.

In any research project, investigators must consider carefully how to safeguard confidential information (including protected health information); this responsibility applies equally to data collected using PDAs. At a minimum, the PDA should be password protected, and collected data should be removed from the PDA as soon as possible. The Health Insurance Portability and Accountability Act (HIPAA, also known as the "Privacy Rule") of 1996, implemented in April 2003, is a federal rule that addresses privacy standards for the use and disclosure of individually identifiable health information. It applies to research data held in electronic form as well, and researchers should be knowledgeable about the federal HIPAA regulations as well as the policies and procedures used by local organizations where nurse researchers are employed. The U. S. Department of Health and Human Services, Office of Civil Rights, has an excellent Web site that explains HIPAA requirements (http://www.hhs.gov/ocr/hipaa/), including a link specifically addressing the Privacy Rule and research.

The availability of technical support is a critical issue when many members of a research team are dependent on the use of the PDA for direct data entry, because there are no hard-copy forms available as backup in the event that the electronic data are lost or corrupted. Members of the research team should have access to computer experts who are knowledgeable about the hardware and software being used, the issues of synchronization and data portability, and the knowledge of how to back up data files on both the PDAs and the base station. If infrared synchronization or wireless transfer of material is being contemplated, issues of network security should be resolved. The convenience of collecting data electronically and not having paper forms to maintain in a secure environment seems attractive, but the potential liability of not having these forms available must be weighed in making the decision to have an entirely paperless data collection system.

SUMMARY

In summary, PDAs are useful tools for research data collection. Advantages include increased accuracy and convenience, portability, and ease in moving data from one program to another. Potential disadvantages include the need for education and training in the new technology. As this technology continues to develop, it will likely become the norm. Increased use will lead to the development of additional software applications for researchers and clinicians.

REFERENCE

Lewis, J.A., & Sommers, C.O. (2003). Personal data assistants: Using new technology to enhance nursing practice. *MCN: The American Journal of Maternal Child Nursing, 28,* 66–71.

Chapter 8

Research Collaboratories: Using Technologies to Advance Science

Diane J. Skiba

Science advances through the process of sharing data, theories, ideas, and results. The scientific paper, published in peer reviewed journals or proceedings, is the preeminent format for advancing collective understanding. Formal gatherings such as invited colloquia, conferences and workshops are also important, as are informal exchanges among peers. In all cases shared information is scrutinized and critiqued. Meritorious work becomes part of the collective understanding, thereby advancing the collective enterprise. (National Research Council, 1993, p. 8)

With the advancement of information and communication technologies, particularly network technologies such as the Internet, there is now another mechanism to "further leverage the entire scientific enterprise" (Wulf, 1993). This mechanism, called a "collaboratory," allows technologies to radically enhance the efficiency and effectiveness of research productivity. The word "collaboratory," first coined by Wulf (1989) is the combination of two concepts, collaboration and laboratory. The concept first appeared in a white paper written by Wulf (1989) for a National Science Foundation invitational meeting held at Rockefeller University in New York. This invitational conference and its associated papers were compiled into an unpublished report (Lederberg & Uncapher, 1989) and served as a basis for the National Research Council's (1993) publication on national collaboratories. The purpose of the invitational conference was to examine the use of information technologies to facilitate scientific research. To view a picture of the contributors of this invitational conference, you can retrieve information from Conway's Web site (http://ai.eecs.umich.edu/people/conway/CollabTech/CollabTechWorkshop.html) that documents this chapter in computer science history.

There are several definitions of the collaboratory concept. The first definition offered by Wulf (1989) is a "center without walls, in which the nation's researchers can perform their research without regard to physical location—interacting with colleagues, accessing instrumentation, sharing data and computational resources, and the accessing of information in digital libraries." This definition, in concept, was a vision for the future and promoted the idea that research endeavors could benefit greatly through the collaboration of the right expertise across disciplines. Allowing researchers to work together in a virtual workspace could not only enhance interdisciplinary research but could facilitate new discoveries. As Wulf (1993) stated, "the single most critical resource for innovation is access to stimulating colleagues, particularly those in different disciplines " (p. 854).

The collaboratory was conceptualized as a tool to foster collaboration among the scientific community. On a conceptual level, collaboration among scientists occurs through various mechanisms such as sharing of data, sharing of instruments, joint authoring of papers, cooperative research across sites, and the rapid dissemination of knowledge throughout the scientific community. When Wulf (1989) first introduced the collaboratory concept, there were several key antecedents in place to foster this vision. First, telecommunications, networked worlds, and the rapid expansion of the Internet permeated the scientific communities. Second, information and communication technologies were expanded to move beyond the traditional single-user, general purpose tools for data gathering, analysis, modeling, storage, and dissemination. Third, the revelation that computing needed to support groups rather than just individuals became the focus of researchers, social scientists, computing professionals, and technologists in the mid-1980s (Skiba, 1993). This emerging area, computer supported collaborative/cooperative work (CSCW), demanded the development of new tools to support group work. CSCW tools, sometimes referred to as groupware, provided a platform to support the work of a group, especially members of a group who were geographically dispersed throughout an organization or across institutions (Skiba, 1994). The intent of the collaboratory concept was that both individual scientists and the entire scientific enterprise would advance through sharing and collaboration. As the National Research Council (1993) summarized,

> "the character of scientific sharing of data, theories, ideas, and results is influenced by both cooperation and competition. Collaboration can be construed as a communal relationship that implies social trust and synergy among participants, with mutual benefit as the result" (p.8).

On an operational level, the National Research Council (1993) further explicated that a collaboratory is a:

> distributed computer system with networked laboratory instruments and data-gathering platforms; tools that enable a variety of collaborative activities; financial and human resources for maintaining, evolving and assisting in the use of computer-based facilities [and] digital libraries that include tools for organizing, describing, and managing data and thus enabling the large scale sharing of data. (National Research Council, 1993, p. 7)

Over time, other operational definitions have evolved and expanded the collaboratory concept. Kouzes, Meyer, and Wulf (1996) refined their operational definition as an "integrated, tool oriented computing and communication system to support scientific collaboration" (p.40). In their thinking, they aptly describe the collaboratory concept as the "village square of the information age" (Kouzes, et al., 1996, p. 40). Henline (1998) and Arias, Eden, Fischer, Gorman and Scharff (2000) simplified their operational definition to include any tools that help researchers work together more easily and effectively. Another operational definition offered from the health care arena defines a collaboratory as "an information technology infrastructure that supports cooperation among individuals, groups, or organizations in pursuit of a shared goal by facilitating interaction, communication and knowledge sharing" (Schleyer, 2001, p.1509).

Despite the various conceptual and operational definitions, several themes emerge to define a collaboratory. These themes focus on:

- Cooperation and collaboration
- Sharing of resources (data, information, knowledge, wisdom, and instrumentation)
- Shared and common workspace
- Communication (synchronous and asynchronous)
- Interactions among people and data sources

- Relationships built upon social trust and synergy
- Shared goals and mutual benefits

EXAMPLES OF SCIENTIFIC COLLABORATORIES

Henline (1998) provided summaries of eight different collaboratory projects in the sciences. Three examples are highlighted to demonstrate the wide variety of scientific collaborations. The first is the collaboratory for Microscopic Digital Anatomy that allows biomedical scientists remote access to a specialized research electronic microscope. Another example is the International Personality Item Pool Collaboratory for the development of psychometric measures to study individual differences. This project allows researchers to share data, cojointly develop new items, reanalyze existing data sets, and disseminate new research findings. The third example is from the Oak Ridge National and the Sandia National Laboratories and represents the development of collaborative visualization infrastructure tools.

The Pacific Northwest National Laboratory's Environmental Molecular Sciences Lab (EMSL) designed a virtual nuclear magnetic resonance (NMR) facility. This collaboratory allows access to the NMR spectrometers as well as access to a customized electronic laboratory notebook. This notebook allows "Web-based access to group notes, experimental parameters, proposed molecular structures and other aspects of the research project" (Keating, et al., 2000, p. 172). The project also employs the use of real-time video-conferencing, remote access to shared instruments, and real-time computer display sharing. An evaluation of this project demonstrated the successful use of the virtual NMR to conduct an experiment on heat shock factor protein. The evaluation demonstrated the convenience and efficiency of conducting these experiments. It also identified revisions to the software components that could increase efficiency and effectiveness.

Another example is the Southeast Collaboratory for Structural Genomics, a networked center connecting five institutions: Universities of Georgia, Alabama at Birmingham, Alabama at Huntsville, Georgia State University, and Duke University Medical Center. This collaboratory aims "to develop, integrate, and test all the constituents for carrying out low cost effective and HTP structural genomics research for both prokaryotic and eukaryotic systems" (Adams, et al., 2003). This collaboratory consists of four working groups (protein production, X-ray crystallography, NMR spectroscopy and bioinformatics). Each working group is responsible for their specific contribution to the overall research goals. The bioinformatics group is responsible for the development of database and data mining toolkits.

Perhaps one of the most notable collections of collaboratory work is being conducted at the University of Michigan. Their work includes collaboratories to support science collaboration (Atmospheric Physics Research, clinical radiology, HIV/AIDS, and brain research) as well as engineering partnerships with several businesses such as Lucent, IBM, and Ford. Extensive descriptions of these various collaboratories and information about the design, development, and evaluations of these projects can be retrieved at their Web site: http://www.scienceofcollaboratories.org.

HEALTH CARE COLLABORATORIES

In health care, several different collaboratory models have evolved over the last decade. One noteworthy model is the InterMed collaboratory created by researchers at Stanford, Harvard, and Columbia's medical informatics laboratories (Shortliffe, et al., 1996). The purpose of this collaboratory was to develop medical information systems using cooperative approaches that could be shared via the Internet. One important shared resource developed by the InterMed Collaboratory was computer-based practice guidelines. In each of the institutions, there was an increased emphasis on the use of Clinical Guidelines as specified by the Institute of Medicine. The InterMed Collaboratory created the GuideLine Interchange Format (GLIF) "to allow the exchange of clinical practice guidelines among institutions and computer-based applications" (Ohno-Machado, et al., 1998, p. 357). Numerous publications (Shortliffe, Patel, Cimino, Barnett & Greenes, 1998; Greenes, Boxwala, Sloan, Ohno-Machado, & Deibel, 1999) have explicated both the conceptual and technical work required for the development of the GLIF. Researchers from McGill University's Cognitive Studies in Medicine (Patel, Allen, Arocha & Shortliffe, 1998) conducted an extensive evaluation of the cognitive processes required to translate a text-based clinical guideline to a shared representation. This comparative study examined the development of GLIF representations of an existing text-based guideline for the management of encephalopathy. Their extensive analysis focused on verbal protocols as a data source across a small group of clinicians at each site. This detailed analysis mapped both the cognitive and perceptual steps an individual took to organize their knowledge and clinical reasoning for the specific problem. Patel et al. (1998) summarized that the analysis yielded differences in structure and content as a function of domain expertise. Differences emerged not only in terms of implicit and explicit knowledge of the domain but there were differences as a result of the GLIF development or technical environment (Patel, et al.). The overall conclusion was that teams consisting of both clinicians with domain expertise and computer scientists who understood computer-based representations should codevelop clinical guidelines. Thus, the InterMed Collaboratory demonstrated a successful research enterprise and is considered an exemplar in medical collaboratories.

Another model was the DHNet project that created an electronic infrastructure to encourage research collaboration among dental hygiene professionals. The DHNet served as an electronic network for the National Center for Dental Hygiene Research. There were several components to the DHNet but the most relevant one was the research collaboratory where users may search the knowledge base, contribute to the knowledge base, communicate with other users and learn about the research priorities and agendas in dental hygiene (Forrest & Koopman, 1998).

In nursing, there are numerous references to the use of collaboratories for educational purposes (Skiba, 1997). The term "collaboratory" was also used to describe the creation of a unique partnership between education and practice at the University of Iowa (Dreher, Everett, & Hartwig, 2001). The partnership was developed to create an infrastructure between the College of Nursing and the Department of Nursing to "generate, disseminate, and apply knowledge for the improvement of nursing practice and patient outcomes" (Dreher, et al., 2001 p. 114). This model conceptualized the collaboratory as a "think tank" for nursing.

The only true research collaboratory in nursing was a model created by Woolery and Yensen (1995). This collaboratory was designed to facilitate the various phases of the research process. The prototype was conceptualized to contain both research development resources and research project management tools. The collaboratory was designed to use the Virtual Nursing College as its initial platform. "Research Development resources included funding sources, consultation services, data acquisition, accessing literature and proposal development tools" (Woolery & Yensen, p. 1351). Tools to be included under the project management side were: budget, data management, data analysis tools, task lists, results reporting, and publishing resources (Woolery & Yensen).

The model served as a basis for the development of a patient-outcomes research project in nursing administration (Goodwin, Turner, Allred & Yensen, 1998).

Ozbolt (October 9, 1999) in her testimony to the National Committee on Vital and Health Statistics Hearings on Medical Terminology and Code Development suggested a research collaboratory be established to further research on standardization of nursing data. She suggested that this collaboratory would allow nursing researchers to share work from their homesites and provide a venue to cocreate an international standard for nursing.

RESEARCH COLLABORATORY REQUIREMENTS

Although limited examples of collaboratories are available in health care, there are numerous others in the sciences and education that are beyond the scope of this chapter. It is obvious that there are many diverse types of collaboratories. They are diverse not only in content but in terms of their goals and their interactions. As Kouzes, Myers, and Wulf (1996) projected, there are four broad categories of interactions: peer-to-peer, mentor-student, interdisciplinary, and producer-consumer. Despite the diversity of existing or prototype collaboratories, there are common requirements highlighted by many in the field. These requirements include both technology and human factors. One very important principle that is clearly explicated is that both technological and sociological requirements are equally important in the creation of a collaboratory.

The National Research Council (1993) identified the following basic requirements of a collaboratory:

- Data Sharing (quick and easy access to data, within and across databases)
- Software Sharing (conveniently share software that supports data analysis, visualization, and modeling)
- Control of remote instruments
- Communicating with remote colleagues using both synchronous and asynchronous mechanisms.

Several years later, Kouzes, Myers, and Wulf (1996) identified other core functions that were required tools in a collaboratory. These core tools include:

- Communication tools that incorporate e-mail, chat functions, and video and audio conferencing
- Shared interactive spaces that incorporate shared computer displays and electronic whiteboards
- Shared electronic notebooks that provide distributed access to data, including data entry, searching, multiuser multimedia annotations, and multimedia graphical displays
- File sharing, remote control of online instruments, computational analysis packages, visualization software, and Web browser synchronization

With the continued development of groupware products, Schleyer (2001) described several additional technical tools required in collaboratories. The first is Web-based collaborative workspaces that provide "one-stop access to all information relevant to the project such as policies, standard operating procedures, directories, archives of all discussions and chats and relevant background materials" (Schleyer, p. 1510). In addition to real-time communication, asynchronous communication methods should include e-mail, discussion groups and newsgroup/listservs. Video, Web-based conferencing, and whiteboards are also considered necessary substitutes for face-to-face meetings and interactions. Two new additional components include online web page markup or coediting documentation tools and automatic notification or push technologies to alert users of new items, events, or articles of interest.

There is also the need to recognize the human computer interface and sociology requirements of any collaboratory. Perhaps these requirements are more difficult to achieve. Technological advances address infrastructure demands but human factors cannot easily be resolved. One human computer interface issue is related to the overall design of a collaboratory. The design needs to be user friendly, cognizant of the users' psychosocial needs, and facilitate interoperability (Kouzes, Myers, & Wulf, 1996). In addition, the National Research Council (1993) recommended the requirement of transparency. A collaboratory must "achieve transparency by treating all tools, databases and participants conceptually as being part of a single system with a uniform set of commands accessible from their desktop" (National Research Council, p. 62). Their report also acknowledged the importance of both the social context and institutional requirements. Individual researcher requirements such as funding, recognition, and tenure plus institutional requirements such as funding, policies, and protection of intellectual property are all part of the social context.

Psychosocial issues, as defined by Kouzes, Myers, and Wulf (1996), include autonomy, trust, sense of place, and attention to ritual. It is particularly important that researchers trust each other before any collaboration can begin. As Myers, Chonacky, Dunning, and Leber (1997) so aptly stated, "collaboration is based on a foundation of trust and friendship derived from non-science interactions such as telling jokes in the coffee room" (p. 117). Virtual environments can create a sense of place but people must be comfortable in those surroundings and work to develop a social presence within the collaboratory. Olson, Teasley, Bietz, and Cogburn (2002) defined three dimensions to assess the readiness for a collaboratory. The first dimension is readiness to collaborate; this is clearly the most basic prerequisite requirement. This dimension includes such broad components as: "motivation to collaborate, shared principles of collaboration and experience with the specific elements of collaboration" (Olson, et al., p. 46). The final two dimensions, collaboration infrastructure and collaboration technology readiness, focus on aspects such as technology support, bandwidth, and training, to work with technologically sophisticated tools. It is certainly one thing to send e-mail and it is another issue to participate in a synchronous whiteboard discussion with coediting facilities. There is no doubt that without a sufficient level of readiness in all three dimensions it would be difficult to have a collaboratory concept succeed and be sustained over time. User-centered design and the inclusion of behavioral scientists in the creation of collaboratory can insure proper attention to the human elements (Finholt, 1995). In summary, both technical and human factor elements must be present to achieve a successful and sustainable research collaboratory.

SUMMARY

Technological advances continue to push the traditional research paradigm. Many consider the collaboratory concept as an emerging research alternative to be both an opportunity and a challenge. The collaboratory concept is built upon several principles. First, it allows researchers to work collaboratively regardless of location. Second, it allows researchers to share resources such as people, ideas, theories, data, and instruments. Third, it allows researchers to reach shared research goals, derive mutual benefits, and collectively solve the most pressing research questions in health care. In Zerhouni's (April 2, 2003) Opening Statement on the Fiscal Year 2004 President's Budget Request, he echoes these ideas and supports the research collaboratory principles. In particular, two of these three themes for the future of NIH research include the changing dynamics of research teams and the need to reengineer the national clinical research enterprise. Fourth, there are definite technology and human factor requirements of any collaboratory. Careful attention to the psychosocial needs of the researcher within these virtual environments should be an integral part of the design of any collaboratory. These human factor elements must be addressed before exploiting the numerous opportunities afforded by emerging and cutting-edge information and communication technology advances. Lastly, shared research goals coupled with economic and societal demands are driving forces to foster collaborative research. For nursing, collaboratories provide an extraordinary opportunity to transform the research enterprise and encourage collaborative endeavors across disciplines, institutions, and countries. To achieve this opportunity, it will be necessary for nursing to begin the "fundamental transformation of scientific practice at the social level" (Teasley & Wolinsky, 2001 p. 2255).

REFERENCES

Adams, M., Dailey, H., DeLucas, L., Lun, M., Prestegard, J., Rose, J., et al., (2003). The Southeast Collaboratory for Structural Genomics: A high-through-put gene to structure factory. *American Chemical Society Research, 36,* 191–198.

Arias, E., Eden, H., Fischer, G., Gorman, A., & Schraff, A. (2000). Transcending the individual human mind—creating shared understanding through collaborative design. *Association of Computing Machinery Transactions in Computer-Human Interaction, 7,* 84–113.

Dreher, M., Everett, L., & Hartwig, S. (2001). The University of Iowa Nursing Collaboratory: A Partnership for creative education and practice. *Journal of Professional Nursing, 17,* 114–120.

Finholf, T. (1995). Evaluation of electronic work: Research on Collaboratories at the University of Michigan. *Special Interest Group: Office Information Systems Bulletin, 16*(2), 49–51.

Forrest, J., & Koopman, A. (1998). DHNet: A model for international research collaboration. *Journal of Allied Health, 27,* 39–44.

Goodwin, L., Turner, B., Allred, C., & Yensen, J. (1998). A virtual patient outcomes research collaboratory for nurse administrators. In. S. Moorhead & C. Delaney (Eds.), *Series on nursing administration: Information systems innovations for nursing* (Volume 10, pp. 30–47). Thousand Oaks, CA: Sage.

Greenes, R. A., Boxwala, A., Sloan, W. N., Ohno-Machado, L., & Deibel, S. R. (1999). A framework and tools for authoring, editing, documenting, sharing, searching, navigating, and executing computer-based clinical guidelines. *Proceedings of the American Medical Informatics Association,* 261–265.

Henline, P. (1998). Eight collaboratory summaries. *Interactions, 5,* 66–72.

Keating, K., Myers, J., Pelton, J., Bair, R., Wemmer, D., & Ellis, P. (2000). Development and use of a virtual NMR facility. *Journal of Magnetic Resonance, 143,* 172–183.

Kouzes, R. T., Meyer, J. D, & Wulf, W. A . (1996). Collaboratories: Doing Science on the Internet, *IEEE Computer, 29*(8), 40.

Lederberg, J., & Uncapher, K. (1989). *Towards a national collaboratory: Report of an invitational workshop at the Rockefeller University, March 17–18. Rockefeller University Collaboratory Workshop.* Washington, DC: National Science Foundation, Directorate for Computer and Information Science Engineering.

Myers, J., Chonacky, N., Dunning, T., & Leber, E. (1997). Collaboratories: Bringing National Laboratories into the Undergraduate Classroom and Laboratory via the Internet. *Council on Undergraduate Research Quarterly, 17,* 116–120.

National Research Council (U.S.), Committee on a National Collaboratory: Establishing the User-Developer Partnership. (1993). *National collaboratories: Applying information technology for scientific research.* Washington, DC: National Academy Press.

Ohno-Machado, L., Gennari, J., Murphy, S., Jain, N., Tu, S., Oliver, D., et al. (1998). The Guideline Interchange Format: A model for representing guidelines. *Journal of the American Medical Informatics Association, 5,* 357–372.

Olson, G. M., Teasley, S. D., Bietz, M., & Cogburn, D. (2002). Collaboratories to support distributed science: The example of international HIV/AIDS research. *Proceedings of the 2002 annual research conference of the South African institute of computer scientists and information technologists on enablement through technology* (pp. 44–51). Republic of South Africa: South African Institute for Computer Scientists and Information Technologists.

Ozbolt, J. (1999, October 19,). *Testimony to the National Committee Center for Vital Health Statistics Hearings on Medical Terminology and Code Development.* Retrieved July 5, 2003, from http://www.mc.vanderbilt.edu/nursing/informatics/ pdf/NCVHSTest10_99.pdf

Patel, V. L., Allen, V., Arocha, J., & Shortliffe, E. (1998). Representing clinical guidelines in GLIF: Individual and Collaborative experience. *Journal of the American Medical Informatics Association, 5,* 467–483.

Science of Collaboratories. Retrieved July 5, 2003, from http://www.scienceofcollabortories.org

Schleyer, T. K. L. (2001). Collaboratories: Leveraging information technology for cooperative research. *Journal of Dental Research, 80,* 1508–1512.

Shortliffe, E. H., Patel, V. L., Cimino, J., Barnett, O.G., & Greenes, R. A. (1998). A study of collaboration among medical informatics research laboratories. *Artificial Intelligence in Medicine, 12,* 97–103.

Shortliffe, E. H., Barnett, O. G., Cimino, J., Greenes, R. A., Huff, S. & Patel, V. L. (1996). Collaborative medical informatics research using the Internet and the World Wide Web. *Proceedings of the American Medical Informatics Association Annual Fall Symposium,* 125–129.

Skiba, D. (1997). The learning collaboratory: A knowledge building environment for nursing education. In U. Gerdin, M. Tallberg, & P. Wainwright (Eds.), Nursing informatics: The impact of nursing knowledge on health care informatics. *Proceedings of the Sixth International Conference.* Amsterdam, Netherlands: IOS Press.

Skiba, D. (1994). Shared knowledge using collaborative tools. *Reflections, 20*(2), 16–18.

Skiba, D. (1993). Collaboration tools. *Reflections, 19*(1), 10–12.

Teasley, S., & Wolinsky, S. (2001). Communication. Scientific collaborations at a distance. *Science, 292,* 2254–2255.

Woolery, L., & Yensen, J. (1995) Nursing collaboratory development via the Internet. Medinfo '95. P*roceedings of the 8th World Congress on Medical Informatics* (pp. 1349–1352). North-Holland, Vancouver, Canada.

Wulf, W.A. (1989). The national collaboratory—a white paper. In J. Lederberg & K. Uncaphar (Eds.), *Towards a national collaboratory: Report of an invitational workshop at the Rockefeller University, March 17–18, 1989* (pp. Appendix A). Washington, DC.: National Science Foundation, Directorate for Computer and Information Science Engineering.

Wulf, W. A. (1993). The collaboratory opportunity. *Science, 261,* 854–855.

Zerhouni, E. A. (2003, April 2,). Opening Statement on the FY 2004 President's Budget Request. Retrieved July 5, 2003, from http://www.nih.gov/about/director/budgetrequest/FY2004budgetrequest.htm

Chapter 9

Survey Research

Eun-Shim Nahm, Mary Etta C. Mills, and Barbara M. Resnick

The Internet began in the late 1960s as a way of linking several universities and defense laboratories. Until 10 years ago, the Internet was available to only a small number of computer users (Moschovitis, Poole, Schuyler, & Senft, 1999). The number of the Internet users, however, has grown exponentionally since the World Wide Web (WWW or "the Web") emerged in 1991. The strength of the Web is easy access to the Internet using predominantly a graphical interface to information (Dix, Finlay, Abowd, & Beale, 1998). As of September 2001, 143 million Americans (about 54% of the population) reported using the Internet (U. S. Department of Commerce, Economics and Statistics Administration, and National Telecommunications and Information Administration, 2002).

As the number of Web users increases, researchers' interest in the Web as a research medium has also grown (Buchanan & Smith, 1999; Duffy, 2002; Witmer, Colman, & Katzman, 1999). For example, Web experimental studies in psychology are becoming increasingly popular (Birnbaum, 1999; Reips, 1995; Smith, & Leigh, 1997), and Web surveys have been undertaken in many areas, such as business (Grossnickle & Raskin, 2001) and health care fields (Duffy, 2002; Hollowell, Patel, Bales, & Gerber, 2000; Houston & Fiore, 1997; Klapper, Klapper, & Voss, 2000).

Specifically, the emergence of electronic surveys has been identified as one of the revolutionary advances in survey history during the 20th century (Dillman, 2000). For both methodological and economic reasons, electronic surveys are attracting considerable interest. Researchers, however, have also raised some methodological issues, such as data validity, sample representativeness, duplicate submission, and missing data (Krantz & Dalal, 2001; O'Neil & Penrod, 2001; Schmidt, 1997). Until recently, Web studies in the academic arena have focused only on college students (Bailey, Foote, & Throckmorton, 2000; Joinson, 1999) and on active professionals, such as health care providers (Houston & Fiore, 1997; Schleyer & Forrest, 2000).

The purpose of this chapter is to provide a brief overview of the development of Web surveys and their advantages and the methodological issues based on the authors' previous research and findings from the literature.

DEVELOPMENT OF WEB SURVEYS

A Web survey can be created using various programming languages, Web page development programs, or commercial Web survey programs. A program will be selected based on the complexity level of the Web questionnaire and available resources. Researchers need to consider the following factors: (a) interactivity, (b) built-in skip patterns and error checking systems, (c) method for submitting responses, (d) data storage, and (e) use of security measures. In addition, researchers will need to have some idea of the types and versions of computers and Web browsers that will be used by potential participants. Generally, it is advisable to develop a Web survey that works for even the lowest-end operating systems and Web browsers.

Developing Web Questionnaires Using Programming Languages

To develop Web questionnaires using programming languages, developers often use Hypertext Markup Language (HTML) or HTML with Java or JavaScript (Baron & Siepman, 2000; Gosselin, 2002). HTML documents are plain-text files that can be created using any text editor (e.g., SimpleText on a Macintosh or Notepad on a Windows®-based computer). JavaScript enhances the static HTML Web page as an interactive Web page. For example, it allows the participant to enter answers on the questionnaire that appears on Web pages. The JavaScript language first became available in the Web browser Netscape Navigator® 2. Later, Microsoft® added its own brand

JavaScript to Internet Explorer,® which they named JScript. Since then, both Netscape® and Microsoft®5 have released improved versions and included them in their latest browser. Therefore, the developers of Web questionnaires need to be aware that these different brands and versions may be incompatible with different browsers. Java programming language is completely different from JavaScript. Essentially, Java can create the same programs that JavaScript can, but it is a more powerful programming language (Gosselin). One of the most efficient features of Java is its architecturally neutral program; therefore, it works on different types of browsers (Tittel & Gaither, 1995).

To send the data entered to the Web questionnaire which was developed using programming languages to a usable database in a server, a Common Gateway Interface (CGI) script needs to be written. The CGI script can be written using various programming languages: JavaScript or Perl, for example (Brenner & Aoki, 1996).

Developing Web Questionnaires Using Web Server

Completing a Web questionnaire is a dynamic process between a participant's computer and the Web server. Therefore, researchers who conduct Web surveys need basic knowledge about the Web server that participants will use. A Local Area Network (LAN) administrator or an administrator of the server should to be consulted before creating a Web questionnaire.

The Web is based on a client-server model in which a client requests services and a server provides resources (Budnick, 1996). On the Web, thousands of servers are in use. All are accessible to browsers using a common protocol, the Hypertext Transfer Protocol (HTTP). HTTP is based on an exchange of requests and responses (Brenner & Aoki, 1996). Many HTTP servers, however, do little more than obtain and send pre-existing files to a client. These HTTP servers have not been designed for complex data processing, such as retrieving information from a database or searching through text fields.

One way to add features for data processing to the HTTP servers would be to make modifications to the server program itself. This process, however, is rather complex and requires detailed knowledge about the server. Therefore, most HTTP servers use a less direct approach. The server does not perform the work itself. Instead it delegates complex tasks to an external program or script (e.g., CGI script). For example, in the case of database access, the script acts as a gateway between the server and the data repository. When the server receives a request to access a database, it passes the request to a gateway program that processes the data and returns the results to the server. The server then returns this information to the client.

Developing Web Questionnaires Using Software Programs

With rapidly advancing technology, researchers can easily create simple Web surveys without the need to learn programming languages. One way is to use the Microsoft FrontPage® and Access database® programs to create Web surveys. Both programs are included in the Microsoft Office® program; therefore, no additional funds are needed to purchase specific programs to develop a Web questionnaire. A questionnaire can be developed using the *Form* function of FrontPage® and saved as an Active Server Page (ASP). An ASP is an HTML page that includes one or more scripts that are processed on a Microsoft Web server before the page is sent to the user.

In addition, the FrontPage® *form* function has the capability of creating an Access® database in the Microsoft Web server to store the data from the users. Unfortunately, however, there are some limitations in assigning variable names and data formats in this automatic process. To overcome this limitation, researchers can add their own Access® database and establish a link between the Web questionnaire and the database in the server. To create a pop-up screen, accuracy check, or skip patterns, Java or JavaScript needs to be added to the program.

Another commercial program that is often used by researchers is the FileMaker Pro 6 Unlimited program (http://www.filemaker.com/ products/ fmu_home.html). This database can accommodate more data and more concurrent users than Access®.

Academic researchers have developed several survey-generating programs that can be used free for academic research: *SurveyWiz* by Michael H. Birnbaum (http://www.governet.net/surveywiz, Birnbaum, 2000) and WWW Survey Assistant by William Schmidt (http://or.psychology.dal.ca/~wcs/hidden/home.html, Schmidt, 1997). Various commercial programs have the capabilities of both creating Web surveys and analyzing data. Table 9.1 shows a few examples of such programs and their Web sites. Costs for these programs vary, based on the number of licenses or the length of the contracted time period.

Table 9.1 Examples of Commerical Web Survey Programs

Advanced Survey Software	http://www.advancedsurveysoftware.com
AskAnywhere®	http://www.senecio.com/askanywhere.html
FormSite	http://www.formsite.com
snap®	http://www.snapsurveys.com/software/softwareprof.shtml
Survey Said™	http://www.surveysaid.com
Survey Select Expert	http://surveyconnect.com
Survey Tracker®	http://www.surveytracker.com/htm/software/software.htm
SurveyMonkey.com	http;//www.surveymonkey.com
Zoomerang™	http://www.zoomerang.com/Login/index.zgi

ADVANTAGES AND METHODOLOGICAL ISSUES

Advantages

Easy access to a demographically and culturally diverse participant population. Although types of sample characteristics depend on the purpose of a study, the globally connected Web provides researchers with vast opportunities to reach out to various populations. For example, researchers can readily conduct culturally specific studies (Barry, 2001), studies of rare diseases (Fyfe, Leonard, Gelmi, Tassell, & Strack, 2001), or studies dealing with specific populations (Finn, 2000; Goritz & Schumacher, 2000; Klapper, Klapper, & Voss, 2000; Sell, 1997).

Cost efficiency. Web surveys eliminate any significant costs for paper, postage, and mailing (Dillman, 2000). The cost for coding data can also be eliminated by linking the Web surveys with the databases directly (Dillman; Houston & Fiore, 1997). Based on the findings from a study of 450 dental professionals (Schleyer & Forrest, 2000), the cost of the Web-based survey was 38% less than that of an equivalent mail survey.

Reduction in cost, however, has to be balanced against the possible need for additional resources depending on the sophistication of the questionnaire design, the level of security that the research requires, and the resources the researcher already has. When researchers have the capability of creating their own survey and have access to a secure server, costs can be minimized. Many researchers, however, do not have these resources. In these instances, the cost of conducting a complex Web survey project can exceed that of the traditional mail survey. In addition, maintaining a high security level can be costly for the researcher, depending on the available network environment.

   Time efficiency and time convenience. Once Web surveys are posted on the Web and announced through appropriate channels (e.g., supporting Web pages, new groups, electronic mailing lists, or various search engines), data collection is almost instantaneous. Unlike traditional surveys, there is no time delay for mailing and returning paper-based questionnaires. In addition, participants are given the opportunity to complete the survey at their own convenience and pace. It has been reported that respondents are more disclosing and direct on electronic surveys than traditional surveys (Joinson, 1999; Kiesler & Sproull, 1986; McKenna & Bargh, 1998).

   Completely voluntary participation. Participants in Web surveys are more active, as they need to seek out and complete the surveys by themselves. Therefore, the risk of coerced participation is minimized (Buchanan & Smith, 1999; Houston & Fiore, 1997; Reips, 2000).

   Efficient data entry. The data that respondents enter can be automatically directed and populated to statistical databases designed by the researcher. Coding and data entry processes can be completely eliminated (Dillman, 2000; Houston & Fiore, 1998; Reips, 2000). Data entry error may also be eliminated. Skip patterns of the questionnaire can be incorporated in Web surveys to direct participants to the right section of the survey, based on their responses. As participants enter responses, the validity of data can be examined on Web surveys (Baron & Siepmann, 2001). For example, if participants entered invalid data (e.g., out-of-range data), a pop-up screen can alert them to enter valid data.

   Capability of adding multimedia. Using Web surveys, a nearly infinite variety of shapes and colors can be used to format a particular survey. Pictures or audios can be easily incorporated into a Web survey. Multimedia functions, however, need to be used judiciously. Participants might have difficulty downloading Web pages or might not have programs to run the multimedia features (e.g., plug-in programs).

Methodological Issues

Sample. Current users of the Web do not necessarily represent the overall total population or desired sample. Although a large number of Americans have access to the Web, only 54% of Americans (143 million) use the Internet on a regular basis, and the majority of online users are still young adults (U.S. Department of Commerce et al., 2002). Among the overall population, 60% of Internet users are Caucasian, and the majority of the users report some college education and higher incomes (U.S. Department of Commerce et al.). More importantly, due to lack of accessibility, underserved populations might not be represented.

Web respondents are a self-selected group, which could result in biased findings (Dillman 2000; Houston & Fiore, 1997; Kaye & Johnson, 1999; Reips, 2000). For instance, only those comfortable with completing Web surveys are likely to participate. To help prevent this type of bias, a researcher can offer both paper- and Web-based surveys in their projects. In many Web surveys, designing random sampling is difficult because often a sampling frame is not available (Brenner & Aoki, 1996; O'Neil & Penrod, 2001; Reips).

Response rate. Calculation of response rates for Web surveys can be difficult unless researchers use e-mail to solicit participation or other means such as recruiting subjects face-to-face or via U.S. mail. Often, however, Web surveys are announced directly on the Web, and the visitors to the Web site decide whether to participate in the posted study or not. In these instances, the researcher could install a counter tracking device to determine how often the Web site is accessed. These counters, however, do not guarantee that a visitor read the study, nor can they distinguish repeated calls from the same visitors (Smith & Leigh, 1997). Another method to keep track of the number of visitors is using server activity logs that include information about each visitor's Internet Protocol (IP) address (Smith & Leigh). An IP address, however, does not always serve as a user's unique identifier. For instance, a number of visitors from one proxy server can have the same IP address, or several people who use the same computer in a computer lab can have the same IP address. Therefore, in this case, calculation of response rates cannot yield valid data. Response rates can also vary.

Informed consent. The increased use of the Web in research has heightened concerns about informed consent. In the past, consent to participate in Web surveys was often taken for granted because participation was completely voluntary (Fischbacher, Chappel, Edwards, &

Summerton, 2000). Web surveys, however, must be approved by the researchers' Institutional Review Board (IRB) and informed consent from participants must be obtained (Goodman, 2000; Houston & Fiore, 1997; Karlinsky, 1998; Robinson, 2001).

Security. Although the HIPAA Security Rule will be effective beginning April 21, 2005 (http://a257.g.akamaitech.net/7/257/2422/14mar20010800/edocket.access.gpo.gov/2003/pdf/03–3877.pdf), ensuring security of data is one of the primary concerns in Web surveys. Various levels of security can be implemented; however, maintaining a high level of security is costly. Researchers need to decide the appropriate level of security required for their research.

Technical issues. Sophistication and user friendliness of the Web survey design depend on resources available and the capability of the researcher. In addition, compatibility among Web survey programs, Web browsers (types and versions), and the type of computer operating systems need to be carefully examined and tested before the Web is actually used (Baron & Siepman, 2001; Schmidt, Hoffman, & MacDonald, 1997). For example, some functions, such as skip patterns, might work for Microsoft Internet Explorer® but not for Netscape Navigator,® or vice versa.

Psychometric aspects of Web questionnaires. To assess certain psychosocial attributes (e.g., social support, quality of life) with Web-based questionnaires, researchers have often used existing instruments either with the same questions as in paper-based questionnaires or with items modified for Web surveys (Buchanan, 2000; Davis, 1999; Soetikno, Provenzale, & Lenert, 1997; Wright, 2000). Unfortunately, only a few researchers reported psychometrics for the Web version of these instruments (Buchanan; Davis). Lack of rigor in measurement in Web surveys still exists.

Procedures. Web surveys can be conducted using various designs. Often, multiple contacts yield a higher response rate (Dillman, 2000). This method, however, is only applicable when the researcher can reach respondents via e-mail, U.S. mail, or telephone. In some Web surveys, researchers might not have respondents' contact information.

When a survey is posted on an organizational Web site, organizational support can increase the response rate. For instance, an announcement of the Web survey with a direct link can be included in members' electronic newsletters. If the study is posted on a researcher's own Web page, the study should be announced in various Internet search engines, appropriate discussion groups, or mailing lists, if possible.

Analysis. In Web surveys, data submitted by participants can be directly populated to a designated database. Researchers must carefully examine data to identify any invalid, duplicate, or missing items. Researchers may need to develop guidelines for data cleaning. For example, Web surveys do not prevent entry of malicious data, such as all "0"s or "1"s (although some questionnaires can have all "0"s or "1"s as valid answers) (Houston & Fiore, 1997). Data from these records will need to be excluded from the analysis.

Web surveys can be particularly vulnerable to duplication (Kaye & Johnson, 1999). Duplication can occur when a respondent inadvertently clicks the submit button more than once. These duplications can be detected in the database, since duplicated records will have the same data and IP address, and are sent within one or two minutes.

In interpreting data, researchers need to consider sample bias. Web users are often demographically skewed, and participants of Web surveys are self-selected groups. Therefore, researchers need to be careful in generalizing findings from Web surveys to larger populations.

SUMMARY

With the increased number of Web users and the advancement of technology, Web surveys are drawing significant attention from researchers. Due to global connectivity and unbounded geographic limitation, Web surveys provide the following advantages: (a) cost and time efficiency, (b) convenience, (c) completely voluntary participation, (d) efficient data entry, and (e) multimedia capabilities.

Web surveys, however, include several inherent methodological issues: (a) sample bias, (b) difficulty obtaining a randomized sample, (c) difficulty in calculating response rates, (d) issues of informed consent and the compliance with the HIPAA Privacy Rule, (e) concerns about the reliability and validity of instruments used in Web surveys, and (f) ongoing data security issues. In addition, cost efficiency is often listed as one of the advantages of Web surveys; however, depending on the sophistication of the Web survey, available resources, and level of security, the ultimate cost of a Web survey can surpass that of a mail survey.

As technology advances, more individuals will use the Web in the near future. Consequently, Web surveys offer many opportunities to conduct research. Researchers, however, must be aware of benefits and pitfalls of Web surveys to achieve desired outcomes.

REFERENCES

Bailey, R. D., Foote, W. E., & Throckmorton, B. (2000). Human sexual behavior: A comparison of college and Internet surveys. In M. H. Birnbaum (Ed.), *Psychological experiments on the Internet* (pp. 141–168). San Diego, CA: Academic Press.

Baron, J., & Siepman, M. (2001). Techniques for creating and using Web questionnaires in research and teaching. In M. H. Birnbaum (Ed.), *Psychological experiments on the Internet* (pp. 235—265). San Diego, CA: Academic Press.

Barry, D. T. (2001). Assessing culture via the Internet: Methods and techniques for psychological research. *CyberPsychology & Behavior, 4*(1), 17–21.

Birnbaum, M. H. (1999). Testing critical properties of decision making on the Internet. *Psychological Science, 10*, 399–407.

Birnbaum, M. H. (2000). SurveyWiz and FactorWiz: JavaScript Web pages that make HTML forms for research on the Internet. *Behavior Research Methods, Instruments, and Computers, 32*, 339–346.

Brenner, S. E., & Aoki, E. (1996). *Introduction to CGI/Perl*. New York: M & T Books.

Buchanan, T. (2000). Internet research: Self-monitoring and judgments of attractiveness. *Behavior Research Methods, Instruments, & Computers, 32*, 521–527.

Buchanan, T., & Smith, J. L. (1999). Using the Internet for psychological research: Personality testing on the World Wide Web. *British Journal of Psychology, 90*, 125–144.

Budnick, L. (1996). *The Windows NTTM Web Server Book*. Research Triangle Park, NC: Ventana.

Davis, R. N. (1999). Web-based administration of a personality questionnaire: Comparison with traditional methods. *Behavior Research Methods, Instruments, & Computers, 31*, 572–577.

Dillman, D. A. (2000). *Mail and Internet surveys: The tailored design method*. New York: John Wiley & Sons.

Dix, A., Finlay, J., Abowd, G., & Beale, R. (1998). *Human-computer interaction* (2nd ed.). London: Prentice Hall Europe.

Duffy, M. E. (2002). Methodological issues in Web-based research. *Journal of Nursing Scholarship, 34*, 83–88.

Finn, J. (2000). A survey of domestic violence organizations on the World Wide Web. *Journal of Technology in Human Services, 17*, 83–102.

Fischbacher, C., Chappel, D., Edwards, R., & Summerton, N. (2000). Health surveys via the Internet: Quick and dirty or rapid and robust? *Journal of the Royal Society of Medicine, 93*, 356–359.

Fyfe, S., Leonard, H., Gelmi, R., Tassell, A., & Strack, R. (2001). Using the Internet to pilot a questionnaire on childhood disability in Rett syndrome. *Child: Care, Health and Development, 27*, 535–543.

Goodman, K. W. (2000). Using the Web as a research tool. *MD Computing, 17*(5), 13–14.

Goritz, A. S., & Schumacher, J. (2000). The WWW as a research medium: An illustrative survey on paranormal belief. *Perceptual & Motor Skills, 90*(3 Pt 2), 1195–1206.

Gosselin, D. (2002). *JavaScript* (2nd ed.). Canada: CourseTechnology.

Grossnickle, J., & Raskin, O. (2001). *Handbook of online marketing research.* New York: McGraw-Hill.

Hollowell, C. M., Patel, R. V., Bales, G. T., & Gerber, G. S. (2000). Internet and postal survey of endourologic practice patterns among American urologists. *Journal of Urology, 163,* 1779–1782.

Houston, J. D., & Fiore, D. C. (1997). Online medical surveys: Using the Internet as a research tool. *MD Computing, 15,* 116–120.

Joinson, A. (1999). Social desirability, anonymity, and Internet-based questionnaires. *Behavior Research Methods, Instruments, & Computers, 31,* 433–438.

Karlinsky, H. (1998). Internet survey research and consent. *MD Computing, 15,* 285.

Kaye, B. K., & Johnson, T. J. (1999). Research methodology: Taming the cyber frontier—techniques for improving online surveys. *Social Science Computer Review, 17,* 323–337.

Kiesler, S., & Sproull, L. S. (1986). Response effects in the electronic survey. *Public Opinion Quarterly, 50,* 402–413.

Klapper, J. A., Klapper, A., & Voss, T. (2000). The misdiagnosis of cluster headache: A nonclinic, population-based, Internet survey. *Headache: The Journal of Head and Face Pain, 40,* 730–735.

Krantz, J. H., & Dalal, R. (2001). Validity of Web-Based Psychological Research. In M. H. Birnbaum (Ed.), *Psychological experiments on the Internet* (pp. 35–60). San Diego, CA: Academic Press.

McKenna, K. Y., & Bargh, J. A. (1998). Coming out in the age of the Internet: Identity "demarginalization" through virtual group participation. *Journal of Personality and Social Psychology, 75,* 681–694.

Moschovitis, C. J. P., Poole, H., Schuyler, T., & Senft, T. (1999). *History of the Internet: A chronology, 1843 to the present.* Santa Barbara, CA: ABC-CLIO.

O'Neil, K. M., & Penrod, S. D. (2001). Methodological variables in Web-based research that may affect results: Sample type, monetary incentives, and personal information. *Behavior Research Methods, Instruments, & Computers, 33,* 226–233.

Reips, U. D. (1995). *Experimental psychology lab.* Retrieved June 7, 2002, from http://www.psychologie.unizh.ch/genpsy/Ulf/Lab/WebExpPsyLab.html

Reips, U. D. (2000). The Web experiment method: Advantages, disadvantages, and solutions. In M. H. Birnbaum (Ed.), *Psychological experiments on the Internet* (pp. 89–117). San Diego, CA: Academic Press.

Robinson, K. M. (2001). Unsolicited narratives from the Internet: A rich source of qualitative data. *Qualitative Health Research, 11,* 706–714.

Schleyer, T. K., & Forrest, J. L. (2000). Methods for the design and administration of Web-based surveys. *Journal of the American Medical Informatics Association, 7,* 416–425.

Schmidt, W. C. (1997). World Wide Web survey research made easy with WWW Survey Assistant. *Behavior Research Methods, Instruments, & Computers, 29,* 303–304.

Schmidt, W. C., Hoffman, R., & MacDonald, J. (1997). Operate your own World Wide Web server. *Behavior Research Methods, Instruments, & Computers, 29,* 189–193.

Sell, R. L. (1997). Research and the Internet: An e-mail survey of sexual orientation. *American Journal of Public Health, 87,* 297.

Smith, M. A., & Leigh, B. (1997). Virtual subjects: Using the Internet as an alternative source of subjects and research environment. *Behavior Research Methods, Instruments, & Computers, 29,* 496–550.

Soetikno, R. M., Provenzale, D., & Lenert, L. A. (1997). Studying ulcerative colitis over the World Wide Web. *American Journal of Gastroenterology, 92,* 457–460.

Tittel, E., & Gaither, M. (1995). *Mecklermedia's official Internet world™: 60 minute guide to Java.* Foster City, CA: IDG Books Worldwide.

U.S. Department of Commerce, Economics and Statistics Administration, & National Telecommunications and Information Administration. (2002). *A nation online: How Americans are expanding their use of the Internet.* Retrieved June 14, 2002, from http://www.ntia.doc.gov/ntiahome/dn/index.html

Witmer, D. F., Colman, R. W., & Katzman, S. L. (1999). From paper-and-pencil to screen-and-keyboard. In S. Jones (Ed.), *Doing Internet research: Critical issues and methods for examining the net* (pp. 145–161). Thousand Oaks, CA: Sage.

Wright, K. (2000). Computer-mediated social support, older adults, and coping. *Journal of Communication, 5,* 100–118.

Chapter 10

Specific Challenges in Using the Internet for Research

Jan V. R. Belcher

For nurses involved in research, the Internet holds enormous potential. Literature searches can be accomplished anywhere at any time with laptop computers and wireless technology. Research experts on different sides of the globe can be reached for consultation instantly. Many culturally diverse global populations can be accessed simultaneously. When nurses use the Internet for research, publication, distribution, and data entry costs can be reduced. However, although the potential for using the Internet for research is enormous, nurses must also realize that caution must be exercised in using the Internet for research. This chapter presents specific opportunities and challenges of this use.

One of the first uses of the Internet was by nurses and other health care providers describing health information on the World Wide Web. Diering and Palmer (2001) found that the Internet contained valuable information on urinary incontinence; however critical skills were needed to evaluate the information. In another study, none of 32 Web sites provided complete information to the public about emergency contraception (Latthe, Latthe, & Charlton, 1999). And in a study about carpal tunnel syndrome, Web sites contained limited information of poor value about the condition (Beredjiklian, Bozentka, Steinberg, & Bernstein, 2000). Many Web sites for arthritis appeared to be profit-based sites used for advertising products (Suarez-Almazor, Kendall, Dorgan, 2001).

Regarding Web site readability, Oermann and Wilson (2000) found that the overall reading level of Internet resources on quality of care that were designed for consumers was 9th grade level, when 8th grade level was recommended for the general public.

A second common use of the Internet in nursing research is data collection. Beckman (2002) used a descriptive Internet survey to study the impact of asthma during pregnancy. In a study with older adults, Clark (2002) used a Web page survey and chat room with people 65 years and older. The majority of the older adults used the computer to decrease loneliness. Other studies collected data from nurses. Im and Chee (2003) used the Internet to conduct a cross-sectional pilot study using 19 participants who were oncology nurse experts in 10 countries. The participants completed a survey on cancer patients and took part in international e-mail group discussions through a Web site and e-mail.

Nurses have also begun to use the Internet for intervention research. On-line support groups are strategies that nurses have been using for interventions. Klemm et al. (2003) reviewed nine research articles that focused on online cancer support groups. They concluded that, even though the samples were small and mostly focused on Caucasian women with breast cancer, the online groups helped people cope with cancer. Participants received both psychological and social support, especially using information seeking and giving. Pierce, Steiner, and Govoni (2002) used online surveys and e-mail discussions to support caregivers of survivors of stroke ($n = 5$). At the end of 3 months, caregivers were generally satisfied with the program and stated they gained information about stroke from the clinical nurse specialist and online Web sites.

SAMPLING CHALLENGES

For research conducted on the Internet, nurses can sample global populations and reach broader untapped populations. Subjects may be more open to discuss confidential topics on the Internet than in a personal interview or with paper and pencil surveys because they have the illusion of anonymity (Burgess, Donnelly, Dillard, & Davis, 2001) and have interactive communication. The interactive communication can be synchronous, that is, several people on the Internet at the same time communicating simultaneously. Communication can also be asynchronous, where a person can post a question anytime, anywhere, and then some-one else answers the question in another time, at another place.

For a convenience sample, nurses can post a survey and invite subjects to participate. Subjects may be selected based on their list-ing in databases, such as using members of an organization, a list-serv, or a chat room. The survey can also be posted on a Web page explaining the research and researchers' qualifications. Sub-jects can then access the survey through listservs, search engines, and even advertisements through publications directing them to the Web site. One study (Burgess et al., 2001) first posted a Web page for potential respondents and then e-mailed the survey to peo-ple who requested the survey. Later, they found that they were receiv-ing too many requests, which were time consuming to process and respond to, and finally posted the survey via a hyperlink on their research Web page. Potential respondents could then download the survey themselves.

Internet sampling can be quicker and more economical than either mailing questionnaires or telephone calls. Mail surveys can take 4–6 weeks and telephone surveys can take from 2–3 weeks as compared to Web-based surveys in 2–3 days (Duffy, 2002). A sample can be larger because it costs less to duplicate the survey and is accessible to populations around the world that might otherwise not be reached by the researcher. However, because respondents may be from around the world, the researcher must be aware of different linguistic and polit-ical orientations. Burgess et al. (2001) found that some respondents had difficulty interpreting survey questions created for a U.S. popula-tion and suggested creating two versions of the survey, one for the U.S. population and one for international respondents.

Another challenge of Internet research is that many people have intermittent access to the Internet. This further limits the sample to whoever had Internet access at the time of the research project. Issues related to intermittent Internet access may be minimized by sending the survey multiple times and collecting data over an extended period of time to increase ones chances of reaching subjects. In addition, in some settings several individuals may have access to the same com-puter such as computer administrators, family members, or cowork-ers. Multiple individuals could complete and send the survey or may access what the original subject answered. Many people have mul-tiple e-mail addresses, which can create confusion when limiting sub-jects to only one response per e-mail address.

For studies describing information on the Internet, sampling Web sites creates different challenges. One reason for the proliferation of the Internet is its capacity to update information instantly. Since research is a systematic examination of phenomena, the Internet presents difficulty in that it changes often and is often difficult to measure and describe. Some researchers have identified consistent ways of searching the Internet for Web sites. For example, to locate Web sites on depression, Belcher and Holdcraft (2003) entered the word "depression" into a metasearch engine, Dogpile. Web sites that dealt with depression glass, The Great Depression, or commercial sites selling products not focused on depression were then eliminated from the search. The first 10 sites on each search engines were examined for information on depression. All hyperlinks on the Web site were examined.

RANDOMIZATION

On the Internet, randomizing subjects for sample selection creates challenges. When one is able to obtain a list of the target population for potential participation in the research project, an advantage is gained as then the researcher can randomly select members from the list who will be contacted. The survey can then be sent to those randomly chosen subjects. Electronic mail can be used to send reminders.

Another challenge is when a subject responds multiple times to one Internet survey. The researcher needs a unique way of identifying each subject. If the researcher is using a database such as an organizational list of names and e-mails, a unique member number may be helpful. Researchers (Burgess et al., 2001) have suggested having one person filter responses to check for multiple submissions and bogus responses. Multiple submissions may be found by comparing identical demographic information and answers on surveys by a computer statistical program. Bogus answers include items that do not correspond to the question asked or that contain letters or numbers that do not communicate meaningful information.

RECRUITMENT

However subjects are sampled, recruiting subjects is a critical part of the research process. In past studies, the range of subject response has varied, with some studies reporting a low response rate and other studies being surprised by the high international response rate. For low response rates, Im and Chee (2003) suggested giving subjects an electronic gift or electronic money to increase response rate.

Potential subjects can be recruited through the Internet or through outside methods such as television, newspaper, or journal advertisements. When subjects are recruited through the Internet, various communication channels can be used. Listservs, newsgroups, chat rooms, e-mails, hyperlinks, and/or information can be posted on Web pages. Search engines can be used to direct subjects to the survey or when subjects "surf the net." Whenever possible, an introduction to the survey should be sent to the potential participant so he or she can choose whether or not to participate. Spamming or sending unsolicited or repeated e-mails should be avoided.

If a survey is posted on the Internet without any selection criteria, everyone on the Internet potentially has access to the survey. Only self-selected volunteers will complete the survey, which can lead to a biased sample. One approach is to screen possible subjects first, then send the survey to selected subjects. Possible subjects could be screened based on demographic or other criteria. When subjects are prescreened the researcher has more control over who completes the survey.

Another advantage of using the Internet for recruitment is the ability to resend a survey or questionnaire. With Internet access, subjects may access the survey anywhere and at any time. Subjects often misplace the paper and pencil surveys before completing the survey. Internet access allows them multiple times to access the survey and easy return to the researchers.

Burgess et al. (2001) described recruiting 300 U.S. and international respondents on involuntary celibacy online survey. A Web page explaining the research with survey hyperlinks was created and posted for one year. Approximately 14% of the subjects were from the original listserv on the topic. Nearly 25% came from links on the Web page. Another 50% came to the site by "surfing the net" or using an Internet search engine. Almost 11% came by word of mouth or posting on Web discussion groups.

MEASUREMENT

Research conducted on the Internet has the same measurement issues as research conducted without the Internet. Measurement issues can affect the validity and reliability of study findings. In creating surveys, the survey should be pilot tested. The Internet gives the researcher access to respondents who might quickly evaluate the survey. Several researchers have asked a listserv group or a chat room to evaluate a pilot survey. Using the Internet for a pilot study can decrease pilot study time and costs.

An Internet survey tool should be constructed with as much thought as a paper-and-pencil survey. Tests for validity and reliability are imperative. In addition, how the survey is displayed on the Internet is important and is discussed later in this chapter.

For intervention studies using the Internet, caution must be taken when relying on self-report measurements or information. Self-report is of particular concern when health care providers, such as nurses, communicate online where there is no face-to-face contact between provider and participant. If the nurse does not assess the health/medical condition first hand, the participant may omit vital information that is needed to make a correct decision. Participants must be told if they have a health/medical condition that is changing or if they need to see a health care provider for treatment.

The Internet provides a wealth of already measured data and health statistics. Researchers can use publicly available large Internet databases for demographics and healthcare service use information. Some Internet databases are free and others have a fee. Federal and state governments provide large linked databases that can be used by researchers, usually at no cost. Some examples are the Centers for Disease Control (CDC) (www.cdc.gov) and the Agency for Healthcare Research and Quality (AHRQ) (www.ahrq.gov), which includes states' inpatient database (SID) (www.ahcpr.gov/data/hcup/hcupsid.htm). Vast information can be obtained from the databases including data on vital events, health status information, hospital discharge information, healthcare use, and expenditures (Vahey, Corser, & Brennan, 2001).

Researchers can use publicly available databases in several different ways. Large databases can provide a useful comparison for data from a specific study and study data can be benchmarked against the databases. For example, the researcher could compare a study's specific medical diagnosis, length of stay, and cost to a national or state database of medical diagnosis, length of stay, and cost.

Another use for large Internet databases is data mining. Data mining is a rapidly developing new research method that extracts patterns and relationships hidden within the databases. Data mining extracts knowledge from data based on artificial intelligence and statistical techniques through the use of computers. With researcher guidance, the computer program builds models to assist in explaining complex relationships. For healthcare, data mining is being used to predict clinical outcomes such as disease survival rates and health outcomes. Goodwin and Iannacchione (2002) used an internal hospital database to examine women ($n = 20,000$) who were at risk for preterm birth. They examined 1,600 variables and found seven predictor variables. As the result of their study, they cautioned that data mining is dependent upon the quality of the data in the database.

Researchers can also perform secondary analyses with existing Internet databases. Secondary data analysis uses data collected from another study or existing database, which reduces the costs and time of collecting primary data. This analysis uses a different organization of data or statistical analyses to reexamine the data. For example, researchers could examine past health care trends to predict future trends at the Health-care Cost and Utilization Project Web site (http://www.ahcpr.gov/data/hcup/hcupnet.htm).

For descriptive research of Web-based information, measuring Web sites is extremely complex. Information and sites can change rapidly, which creates up-to-date information but creates measurement problems for researchers. Belcher and Holdcraft (2003) studied depression Web sites over three time periods. The first time they attempted to evaluate 86 Web sites for depression using a metasearch engine. They found that 28 Web sites (33%) were duplicate and 9 Web sites (10%) were under construction or could not be rated. So they rated 49 Web sites initially. Three months later, they could rate only 42 (80%) of the original Web sites. One year later, they could only rate 23 Web sites (47%) of the original 49 Web sites because Web sites were missing, under construction, or had deleted information about depression.

THEORETICAL CONSIDERATIONS

Thurmond (2002) examined the use of theoretical frameworks for online education research and found a paucity of studies using theory to guide the research. She suggested the lack of a theory and research link limits applicability of the study and the ability to build comprehensive research. Some theories that could be used in online education research include constructivism, systems theory, outcome theory, and the supportive learning theory (Thurmond). Belcher and Holdcraft (2003) used the Technology Assessment Model created by the U.S. Office of Technology in 1982. However, this theory is very broad and was created to be used with any new technology.

Hobbs (2002) reviewed published computer competency instruments for nurses. He found a lack of consistency in agreement on conceptual definitions and measurements of computer competencies. However, in general, computer-competent nurses needed an understanding of computer technology and a positive attitude toward computers. Theoretical considerations for research on the Internet are in the beginning stages and may even need to be borrowed from other disciplines such computer science.

Other theoretical issues are unique to Internet research. One issue is the instant global communication and potential of reaching previously inaccessible populations. This may not be a major problem in research that is exploratory, descriptive, or theory building related to Internet users (Burgess et al., 2001). However, a self-selected nonrepresentative Internet sample creates unique problems for survey research since the sample may not be representative of global populations.

WEB PAGE DESIGN

For Internet based research, Web pages need to be created for introducing the potential respondent to the study and for creating surveys. Web pages can also be a component of a research intervention such as providing health information or creating hyperlinks for e-mail or group discussions. When designing Web pages, many factors need to be considered. First, respondents are using different types of computers. Different computers have different load times that are influenced by computer processing speed, type of Internet connection, and file size of the Web page (Hrabe, Ismeurt, Long, & Greenberg, 2002). Respondents may become bored with a slowly loading Web site. Surveys may also appear differently on different computers. One study found that the respondents using WebTV had more difficulty with moving around the survey and answering questions than those with computer access (Burgess et al., 2001). For a longer survey, the ability to work on the survey, save the survey, and return to the survey at a later time would be beneficial. Researchers should attempt to keep the survey easy-to-read and easy-to-load, while considering the subject's developmental level and any special needs.

Larger fonts (14 points and higher) are recommended for use with older individuals. Highly contrasted fonts and backgrounds may make the text easier to read (e.g., black type on white backgrounds) (Hrabe et al., 2002).

Web page colors should be carefully chosen (Sproat, 2002) and complex reading should be avoided. Reading a computer screen is tiring and slower than reading a newspaper. Children like fun graphics. Multiple large pictures should be used carefully as they increase computer loading time. Hrabe and colleagues (2002) preferred 12 point Arial fonts and used only a third of the computer screen for horizontal text. Other researchers have suggested that surveys within the body of an e-mail may be answered more frequently than surveys that are sent as e-mail attachments.

Previous research has shown that potential computer users who are inexperienced can master computer skills (Klemm et al., 2003). Pierce et al. (2002) found that caretakers of stroke survivors had some technical difficulties using an online support computer program for the first month, but resolved these difficulties by the third month.

International audiences are another challenge for Web page construction. Researchers studying international audiences need to have an international font because some fonts do not transfer. Im and Chee (2003) suggest using universally readable fonts (Times New Roman, Arial) in universally readable file formats. In addition, researchers need to be aware of cultural differences in using religious images and human body parts (Hrabe et al., 2002).

Burgess and colleagues (2001) found that respondents had more difficulty with questions that asked them to skip another question and go to another questions on their Internet survey than on paper-and-pencil tests. For example, a survey might contain Question 1."Have you ever been treated by a professional health provider for depression? Yes or No" and then "If you answered 'No,' please skip Question 2 and go to Question 3." On the Internet-based survey, respondents had difficulty maneuvering around in the survey as compared to on a paper-and-pencil test where pages could be easily flipped.

Another consideration for Web page construction is accommodating the Internet for a wide audience. The World Wide Web Consortium (2003) suggests guidelines to promote accommodations for Internet users with disabilities (http://www.w3.org). Also, the World Wide Web Consortium suggests making the Internet more accessible to other users such as international and mobile audiences. The guidelines address using text equivalents for images, using graceful transformations between screens and tables, using larger fonts or computer magnifying screens, and highlighting hyperlinks for easy navigation. Since the guidelines are periodically revised, researchers will want to make sure their Web pages incorporate the latest recommendations. For Web page construction expertise, an important member of the research team is an expert who can develop Web pages or an external consultant who has these skills and knowledge to assist the research team.

SUMMARY

The Internet holds enormous potential for nurse researchers. However, the Internet is a unique medium that presents both opportunities and challenges. Some opportunities include accessing culturally-diverse global populations, reducing publication and distribution costs, and instantaneously consulting with research experts from around the globe. Research using the Internet also includes challenges to overcome. Some challenges include locating and recruiting representative samples, generating and adapting theory, and creating Internet intervention strategies for all groups of people.

REFERENCES

Beckmann, C. A. (2002). A descriptive study of women's perceptions of their asthma during pregnancy. *MCN: The American Journal of Maternal/Child Nursing, 27*, 98–102.

Belcher, J. V., & Holdcraft, C. (2003, July). *Repeated measures of depression Web sites: Implications for global nursing.* Paper presentation at the 14th International Nursing Research Congress, Sigma Theta Tau International. St. Thomas, Virgin Islands.

Beredjiklian, P. K., Bozentka, D. J., Steinberg, D. R., & Bernstein, J. (2000). Evaluating the sources and content of orthopaedic information on the Internet. *Journal of Bone & Joint Surgery, American Volume, 82-A*, 1540–1544.

Burgess, E. O., Donnelly, D., Dillard, J., & Davis, R. (2001). Surfing for sex: Studying involuntary celibacy using the Internet. *Sexuality and Culture, 5*(3), 5–30.

Clark, D. (2002). Older adults living through and with their computers. *Computers, Informatics, Nursing, 20*, 117–124.

Diering, C. L., & Palmer, M. H. (2001). Professional information about urinary incontinence on the World Wide Web: Is it timely? Is it accurate? *Journal of WOCN, 1*, 55–62.

Duffy, M. E. (2002). Methodological issues in Web-based research. *Journal of Nursing Scholarship, 34*, 83–88.

Goodwin, L., & Iannacchione, M. (2002). Data mining methods for improving birth outcomes prediction. *Outcomes Management, 6*, 80–85.

Hobbs, S. (2002). Measuring nurses' computer competency: An analysis of published instruments. *Computers, Informatics, Nursing, 20,* 63–73.

Hrabe, D., Ismeurt, R., Long, C., & Greenberg, E. (2002). The ergonomics of Web page design: Planning for success. *Computers, Informatics, & Nursing Plus, 5*(3), 2, 6–7.

Im, E. O., & Chee, W. (2003). Issues in Internet research. *Nursing Outlook, 51,* 6–12.

Klemm, P., Bunnell, D., Cullen, M., Soneji, R., Gibbons, P., & Holecek, A. (2003). Online cancer support groups: A review of the research literature. *Computers, Informatics, & Nursing, 21,* 136–142.

Latthe, M., Latthe, P. M., & Charlton, R. (1999). Quality of information on emergency contraception on the Internet. *The British Journal of Family Planning, 26,* 39–43.

Oermann, M. H., & Wilson, F.L. (2000). Quality of care information for consumers on the Internet. *Journal of Nursing Care Quality, 14*(4), 1–12.

Pierce, L., Steiner, V., & Govoni, A. (2002). In-home online support for caregivers of survivors of stroke: A feasibility study. *Computers, Informatics, & Nursing, 20,* 157–164.

Sproat, S. B. (2002). Principles of Web site development and design: Powerful educational tools. *Journal for Nurses in Staff Development, 18,* 68–72.

Suarez-Almazor, M. E., Kendall, C. J., & Dorgan, M. (2001). Surfing the net— information on the World Wide Web for persons with arthritis: Patient empowerment or patient deceit? *The Journal of Rheumatology, 28,* 185–191.

Thurmond, V. (2002). Considering theory in assessing quality of Web-based course. *Nursing Educator, 27,* 20–24.

Vahey, D. C., Corser, W. D., & Brennan, P. F. (2001). Publicly available healthcare databases for administrative strategic planning. *Journal of Nursing Administration, 31,* 9–15.

World Wide Web Consortium. (2003). *Web content accessibility guidelines 1.0.* Retrieved June 28, 2003, from www.w3.org

Chapter 11

Obtaining Grants for Internet-Based Research Projects

Eun-Ok Im and Wonshik Chee

S eeking funding for Internet-based research projects is often difficult and problematic because using the Internet in research tends to be new and innovative, and has some inherent methodological issues (McCormick, Cohen, Reed, Sparks, & Wasem, 1996). Because of the nature of Internet research with non-face-to-face interactions, Internet research has many methodological disadvantages that traditional research methods do not have. On the other hand, because of its use of computer and communication technologies, Internet research may be viewed positively when the proposal is reviewed in terms of innovation. In this chapter, issues in seeking funding for Internet research and writing a proposal for Internet research are discussed, and suggestions for proposal writing for Internet research are made. First, general types of grants supporting Internet research are described, and potential sources of funding are listed. Then, issues in seeking funding for Internet research are discussed. Also, issues in writing a proposal for Internet research are discussed. Finally, based on the discussion of the issues in seeking funding and writing a proposal for Internet research, suggestions for proposal writing for Internet research are made.

FUNDING SOURCES FOR INTERNET RESEARCH

Usually, the researcher may have one of two purposes for seeking research funding. First, the funding may allow the researcher to conduct a single study that is of immediate concern or interest. Another purpose of seeking funding is to initiate or maintain a career of conducting research. The first purpose is most common among nursing students who are preparing theses and dissertations. Except in unusual circumstances, the person seeking funding for a single study, such as a master's thesis, needs to consider sources of small amounts of support. In most cases, this type of funding will not reimburse for salary and will pay only a portion of the costs of the study. Examples of this type of funding are: the Sigma Theta Tau International (STTI) small grants; the Oncology Nursing Foundation (ONF) small grants; the Association of Women's Health, Obstetrics, and Neonatal Nursing (AWHONN) and the American Nurses Foundation (ANF) research grants. The second purpose is most common among nursing faculty and nurses employed in research positions in health care agencies. The individual planning to continue research activities throughout a career needs to plan a strategy for progressively more extensive funding of research activities (Ingersoll & Eberhard, 1999). The purpose of seeking funding for researchers who plan to conduct Internet studies can be either of these two.

Funding sources for Internet research can be categorized into (a) government agencies, (b) professional organizations, and (c) private foundations similar to those for traditional research. Government agencies include the National Institute of Health (NIH) (http://www.nih.gov), which also comprises specialty institutions such as the National Institute of Nursing Research (NINR), the National Institute of Cancer (NCI), and the National Institute of Aging (NIA) (McCormick et al., 1996). The Agency for Health Care Research Quality (AHRQ) has been funding informatics research for more than 25 years including such public and community health projects as the Computer-Stored Ambulatory Record (COSTAR), which included the development of computer languages such as Massachusetts General Hospital Utility MultiProgramming Systems (MUMPS) (McCormick et al.). Other governmental institutions that have funded informatics research include: The Center for Disease Control and Prevention (CDC), the Department of Agriculture/Extension Service, the Department of Agriculture/Rural Utilities Service, the Health Care Financing Administration (HCFA) Office of Research and Demonstration, the Health Resources and Services Administration—Bureau of Health Professions (HRSA-BHP), Division of Nursing (DON), the Health Resources and Services Administration—Office of Rural Health Policy—Rural Telemedicine Grant Program and Rural Health Outreach Grant Program, the National Library of Medicine—Extramural Grants (NLM), and the Department of Commerce—National Telecommunications and Information Administration—Telecommunication and Information Infrastructure Assistance Program.

The Department of Defense (DOD) is also a good funding source for Internet research, as they have funding mechanisms for innovative ideas (http://cdmrp.army.mil/funding/default.htm).

Funding announcements for the federal government can be found in publications such as the *Federal Register* or at each of the home page sites for governmental agencies. The federal government is the largest contributor to the support of research activities (McCormick et al., 1996; Polit & Hungler, 1999). The two major types of federal funding are grants and contracts (Coley & Scheinberg; McCormick et al.). A grant is assistance given to an organization (or individual) to accomplish its (his/her) stated purposes and objectives (Coley & Scheinberg). A contract represents a procurement or purchase arrangement in which the contracting agency "buys" services from the organization (or individual) to fulfill the contracting agency's obligations or responsibilities (Coley & Scheinberg).

Grants are awarded for proposals in which the research idea is developed by the investigator. One mechanism of grants is for agencies and institutes to issue broad objectives relating to an overall mission. A second mechanism of grants is for an agency to issue program announcements (PA) periodically, which describe new, continuing, or expanded program interests. A third mechanism offers federal agencies a means of identifying a more specific topic area in which they are especially interested in receiving applications by a Request for Application (RFA). Unlike a program announcement, an RFA usually specifies a deadline for the receipt of proposals. These approaches to funding differ from investigator initiated research which is the most common mechanism for research funding.

Contracts are usually responding to a Request for Proposals (RFP), and awarded to only one of the competitors (McCormick et al., 1996). An RFP is issued when an agency identifies the need for a specific study, and details the exact work that the government wants done and the specific problem to be addressed. Since the contract method of securing research support severely constrains the kinds of work in which investigators can engage (the researcher responding to a RFP generally has no latitude in developing the research objectives), most researchers want to compete for grants rather than contracts.

Some professional organizations including the Oncology Nursing Society (http://www.ons.org) and the American Nurses Foundation (http://nursingworld.org) are willing to support Internet studies, especially Internet intervention studies. These organizations are more appropriate for small initial research projects because of the limitations in funding amounts. Private foundations and organizations such as the Robert Wood Johnson (RWJ) Foundation (http://www.rwjf.org/index.jsp) and the Susan Komen Breast Cancer Foundation (http://www.komen.org/) are also good funding sources for Internet studies.

Most private foundations have written guidelines for the submission of proposals that can be obtained through a phone call or letter requesting the guidelines. Private organizations such as philanthropic foundations, professional organizations, and corporations tend to be less rigid in their proposal regulations, reporting requirements, clearance of instruments, and monitoring of progress. Information on private funding can be found through the Foundation Center (http://fdncenter.org). Private funding from professional organizations such as the American Nurses Foundation (ANF) (http://www.nursingworld.org), Sigma Theta Tau International (STTI) (http://nursingsociety.org), and the Oncology Nursing Foundation (ONF) (http://www.ons.org) can be found on their Web sites. Sometimes corporations provide private funding. The Foundation Center publishes a directory called Corporate Foundation Profiles and also provides links through its Web site to a number of corporate philanthropic programs. Community of Science, Inc. (COS) (http://www.cos.com) also provides information on currently available research funding opportunities from federal agencies, professional organizations, and private foundations. Still, detailed information on the requirements and interests of funding agencies should be directly obtained from the organization.

ISSUES IN SEEKING FUNDING FOR INTERNET RESEARCH

Because of the innovative nature of Internet research, there are several issues to consider in seeking funding for such research. Sometimes, the innovative nature of Internet research can also be viewed as a strength of the project, but it also can be viewed as a methodological flaw because the Internet has been inadequately tested and evaluated as a research method/setting. The researcher who plans to conduct an Internet study can apply for funding from currently existing federal and private funding agencies, yet he/she first needs to check about the match between his/her proposed study and the goals and objectives of the funding agency. The match between the proposed study and the objectives/goals of funding agencies is frequently reported to be one of the important factors determining the funding (Coley & Scheinberg, 2000).

Few members of scientific review groups for funding agencies are expert in Internet research. Thus, sometimes these review groups cannot appropriately and accurately review Internet research. Sometimes, reviewers have preconceived biases related to Internet research (e.g., Internet research can result in selection bias which cannot be generalizable to other populations) and very limited knowledge of computer technologies. Therefore, researchers might have difficulty obtaining funding when this situation exists. However, with the number of Internet research projects increasing, funding agencies have begun to invite experts in Internet research and/or informatics to serve as guest reviewers.

It is sometimes difficult to determine if Internet research fits into the currently existing categories of funding. For example, in Susan Komen Breast Cancer Foundation research grant mechanisms, population-specific grants exist. Internet research can be a population-specific study if the funding agency considers the Internet population a specific population. An Internet population can be also viewed as a general group of people whom we can see in a shopping mall or on the street. In that case, Internet research cannot fit into the category of funding. It is critical to check directly with the funding agency regarding the fit of an Internet study that the researcher is proposing.

Internet research might cost more than traditional studies although prior research has indicated that Internet research is inexpensive. Internet research does not require expenses for paper and photocopies, or transportation fees for data collection, and this can be considered a strength of the Internet research (Frandsen, 1997; Kollock & Smith, 1999; Lakeman, 1997). However, Im and Chee (2001) indicated that Internet research can be expensive because of the costs for computer servers, Web site development, and programming. This inconsistency in the expense of Internet research can be an issue when applying for funding. When considering the high cost involved in Internet research, some funding resources from private organizations for small grants might not be appropriate. However, depending on the programming needed for Internet research (e.g., simple web questionnaire, simple presentation of education programs), the cost for Internet research can vary.

ISSUES IN WRITING A PROPOSAL FOR
INTERNET RESEARCH

When considering funding for Internet research, there are several issues to consider when writing the proposal. Proposals are generally evaluated on a number of criteria, including the importance of the research questions, theoretical basis, adequacy of research methods, the availability of appropriate personnel and facilities, and the reasonableness of the budget. In addition, many funding agencies use innovation as a review criterion. In terms of the innovation criterion, Internet studies can be evaluated highly. Yet, researchers need to consider that innovation is not the only criterion to evaluate research proposals, and that Internet studies can be scored low in terms of other criteria, especially the adequacy of research methods, because the Internet has only begun to be tested and validated as a research method.

The protection of human subjects warrants considerable attention because interactions between the researcher and research participants are different from those in traditional research. For example, authenticity of the research participants cannot be easily ensured when using the Internet because face-to-face interactions are not present in Internet research (Kollock & Smith, 1999). Researchers need to provide strategies to ensure authenticity of Internet interactions that will be conducted in their Internet studies. O'Brien (1999) asserted that there is strain between those who view online interaction as an opportunity to perform a variety of perhaps fabricated roles versus those who see cyberspace as a new communication medium between real people. The most contested issue in the history of online communication may be how to establish ways of underscoring real versus fictitious sites so that users can reliably distinguish real authenticity from authentic fantasy. When using the Internet in a research project, this issue of real authenticity and authentic fantasy still exists. Research assumes authentic interactions between researchers and research participants. Yet, in reality, it is questionable how authentic the interactions and the phenomena reported and/or explored through the Internet can be. Security of computer servers and safety of data collected through the Internet can easily raise a red flag in the review of Internet research. Therefore, when writing a proposal for an Internet study, researchers must consider currently available guidelines for the protection of human subjects in electronic transmissions including the Health Insurance Portability and Accountability Act (HIPAA) (Frankel & Siang, 1999; U.S. Department of Health and Human Services, 2001).

Another issue is the potential for selection bias in Internet research. Some reviewers view selection bias in Internet research as a major methodological flaw. According to the tenth survey on Internet users by Georgia Tech Graphics Visualization and Usability Center (1999), 33% of the participants were female; regardless of geographic location, new users (those who have been online for less than a year) were quite gender-balanced with 48.5% being female and 51.5% being male; participants were highly educated with 87.8% having at least some college experience and 59.3% having obtained at least one degree; the average age was around 35 years; participants were predominantly white (87.2%); many Internet users worked in university education (11.6%), information services (6.8%), and software (6.0%); and average household income of the Internet users was $57,300. More recent surveys on Internet users have indicated changing demographics of Internet users (HispanicBusiness.com, 2002; ComputersScope Ltd. and others, 2002). Internet usage among Asian-Americans is greater than that of any other ethnic group, and half of U.S. Hispanics and 33% of African-Americans are now Internet surfers. More and more women are using the Internet: women account for 52% of home Internet users (ComputersScope Ltd. and others). Some researchers expect that in the near future selection bias will not be an issue that Internet researchers need to contend with. However, currently, it is still true that Internet users tend to be young, male, white, educated, and wealthy. Therefore, when writing a research proposal for funding, it is important to assure the reviewers about how the potential selection bias will be adequately and appropriately managed.

Because the Internet is very new as a research method, the validity and reliability of the Internet as a research method/setting have been rarely determined or validated. Therefore, it is important to make it clear why use of the Internet in *your* project will be beneficial to the proposed study and how data quality will be similar to that of traditional research. Researchers should seriously consider including findings on comparisons of Internet research methods with other traditional research methods (e.g., telephone survey, mail survey, interviews, etc) when developing the proposal to be submitted to a funding agency. One should also consider including information on the validity and reliability of the Internet format of any instruments that will be used. This information can come from preliminary studies and/or existing literature.

SUGGESTIONS FOR PROPOSAL WRITING FOR INTERNET RESEARCH

As discussed in the previous sections, Internet research has unique characteristics, which should be adequately and accurately incorporated into any research proposal. We propose the following guidelines for those who wish to develop an Internet research proposal.

Prior to beginning any extensive work, researchers should contact potential funding agencies to check with the program director(s) or grant administrator(s) about interest in the proposed idea. Networking with individuals in funding agencies has been emphasized in traditional research (Alvarez, 1999; Sayer, 1999), and it remains important in Internet research. It is also important to discuss potential hindrances for Internet studies and how reviewers would view an Internet proposal. In addition, if a researcher aims at funding from a private foundation, he/she needs to determine if the proposed idea matches the agency's mission and programs (Coley & Scheinberg, 2000).

Researchers are also encouraged to review a successful proposal before writing their own. Reviewing an actual successful proposal can help the novice researcher understand how all the pieces fit together (Turner, 1999). Proposals funded by the federal government are generally considered to be in the public domain. Therefore, researchers can request a copy of any proposals that were funded by writing to the sponsoring agency. In addition, before writing a proposal, researchers should conduct an Internet search through CRISP (Computer Retrieval of Information on Scientific Projects) (http://crisp.cit.nih.gov/) for projects in their area that were recently funded. CRISP is a searchable database of federally funded biomedical research projects conducted at universities, hospitals, and other research institutions. The database is maintained by the Office of Extramural Research at the National Institutes of Health and includes projects funded by NIH, Substance Abuse and Mental Health Services (SAMHSA), Health Resources and Services Administration (HRSA), Food and Drug Administration (FDA), Centers for Disease Control and Prevention (CDC), Agency for Health Care Research and Quality (AHRQ), and the Office of the Assistant Secretary of Health (OASH). Thus, researchers can use the CRISP interface to search for scientific concepts, emerging trends and techniques, or to identify specific projects and/or investigators.

Researchers who intend to submit an Internet-based proposal must pay careful attention to reviewers' criteria. In most cases, the funding agency provides the researcher with information about the criteria that reviewers will use in making funding decisions (Coley & Scheinberg, 2000; Lindquist, Tracy, & Treat-Jacobson, 1995). Criteria are sometimes very simple consisting of a list of questions. In other cases, the criteria are very specific and include specific grading/scoring scales for each criterion. Typically, governmental funding agencies use a weighting system when reviewing proposals, with various weights or points assigned to each section of the proposal (Coley & Scheinberg, 2000). Researchers should keep in mind that funders are looking for projects that are realistic, have measurable outcomes with a good chance for success, and are ambitious. The proposal will be attractive to funding agencies if the project reaches beyond known boundaries to advance the science (Coley & Scheinberg, 2000).

Researchers need to carefully justify and document their decisions and choices of specific topics, methods, and populations. It is particularly important for Internet projects to carefully articulate in the purpose and specific aims sections why an Internet study design is preferred to conventional research methods (e.g., paper-and-pencil questionnaire, mail survey, telephone survey, interviews) for the proposed study. Researchers may want to emphasize that the Internet provides a rich research setting through synchronous and asynchronous communication channels, and that the Internet allows people in geographically dispersed areas to communicate without long distance travels (Frandsen, 1997; Kollock & Smith, 1999).

In the methods section, researchers will need to convince the reviewers that the Internet provides a valid and reliable approach to study the stated problem. As selection bias may be a concern of reviewers, researchers need to provide statistics on Internet users and make it clear that potential selection bias can be easily prevented through study design, sampling, and recruitment strategies to increase generalizability. For example, in the sampling section, researchers may want to explain how to recruit research participants from the targeted populations without selecting a specific group of the population. Researchers also need to discuss how they will ensure that the sample includes an adequate number of participants across racial/ethnic groups, social class, and educational level.

In the instrumentation section, researchers need to provide psychometrics of the Internet format of the instruments that the researchers plan to use to collect data through the Internet. With the increasing number of Internet researchers, some instruments have already been used in previous research as an Internet format. Therefore, researchers need to contact the author of the instruments first and check for information regarding the psychometrics of the Internet format. The author of the tool may request that findings be shared at the completion of the study. If information on the psychometrics of the Internet format of the instruments is not available, the researcher will need to determine the validity and reliability of the Internet format of the instruments through preliminary studies prior to proposal submission.

In the data collection procedures, researchers need to provide details on the project Web site development process with an overall structure of the site. Details are also needed on how informed consent will be obtained through the Internet and how participants will be reimbursed at the completion of the study. Because obtaining informed consent and reimbursing participation through the Internet are not as simple as in studies using traditional methods (Frankel & Siang, 1999; Im & Chee, 2001; Lakeman, 1997), reviewers might have concerns.

Researchers also need to provide details on data management (e.g., where the data will be saved, which format of files will be used, how to store the files, how to save the data in floppy diskettes and in a locked cabinet, who will have access to the data, and how to prevent any possible intrusions by outsiders [e.g., hacking, virus contamination, etc.] and maintain a higher level of security). Because of security and safety issues related to Internet interactions, reviewers will be more concerned about this process than in studies using traditional data collection methods.

Reviewers frequently give considerable weight to the qualifications of research team members, especially the person who is in the lead role on the project (frequently referred to as the principal investigator or PI). During the proposal development process, researchers should carefully scrutinize the qualifications of the research team, and effectively include consultants to address any gaps in the expertise of the team (Fahs & Anderson, 1995). For Internet research, the team will need to include an expert in project Web site development and management, and computer technologies. Having an expert in computer technologies as a coinvestigator and/or consultant will strengthen the proposal. In addition, when composing the research team, it is necessary to have the right mix of competence. With computer experts, without content experts in the research area, a project team may have difficulty convincing reviewers that the project would be successful. Gaps and weaknesses can often be compensated for by the judicious use of consultants (Fahs & Anderson, 1995).

Critique of the proposal by an outside reviewer prior to submission to an outside funding agency is recommended. A draft should be reviewed by at least one other person, preferably someone with relevant methodologic and substantive strengths in the proposed area of research. If a consultant has been proposed because of specialized expertise that researchers believe will strengthen the study, then it would be advantageous to have that consultant participate in the proposal development by reviewing the draft and making recommendations for its improvement (Fahs & Anderson, 1995; Polit & Hungler, 1999). For Internet studies, critique of the proposal by experts in computer technologies in addition to content experts is necessary. They can provide "cutting-edge" information on computer technologies related to the proposed Internet research and consultations on the content areas that Internet researchers might have missed.

CONCLUSIONS

With the advances in computer technologies and the increase in Internet users, we will likely see additional Internet studies in the near future. As telephone surveys were critiqued in terms of research methodology in the past, Internet research can be critiqued because of its relatively recent introduction to nursing research and because it is a new methodology for which reliability and validity must be established. These problems will likely be resolved in the near future with the almost daily advances in computer technologies. In the future, Internet research will be viewed as a common research method similar to mail and telephone surveys. Internet researchers need to continuously make efforts to deal with potential methodological pitfalls related to Internet research and to write fundable research proposals while incorporating the currently raised issues, including limitations in computer technologies, demographic characteristics of Internet users, and the unique characteristics of Internet interactions.

REFERENCES

Alvarez, M. E. (1999). Grant writing in the home health arena: The proposal. *Home Healthcare Nurse Manager, 3*(2), 24–27.

Coley, S. M., & Scheinberg, C. A. (2000). *Proposal writing* (2nd ed.). Thousand Oaks, CA: Sage.

ComputersScope Ltd. et al. (2002). *NUA Internet surveys*. Retrieved February 3, 2002, from http://www.nua.ie/surveys/

Fahs, P. S., & Anderson, F. R. (1995). Effective use of the research consultant. *Journal of the New York State Nurses Association, 26*(4), 14–17.

Frandsen, J. L. (1997). The use of computers in cancer pain management. *Seminars in Oncology Nursing, 13,* 49–56.

Frankel, M. S., & Siang, S. (1999). *Ethical and legal aspects of human subjects research on the Internet.* Retrieved April 17, 2003, from http://www.aaas.org/spp/dspp/sfrl/projects/intres/main.htm.

Georgia Tech Graphics Visualization and Usability Centre. *GVU's 10th WWW user survey* [online]. Available: http://www.gvu.gatech.edu/user_surveys/survey_1998_10/tenthreport.html

HispanicBusiness.com. (2002). *Study: Hispanic Internet use reaches 50 percent.* Retrieved February 3, 2002, from http://www.hispanicbusiness.com/news/newsbyid.asp?id=6135

Im, E. O., & Chee. W. (2001). A feminist critique on the use of the Internet in nursing research. *Advances in Nursing Science, 23*(4), 67–82.

Ingersoll, G. L., & Eberhard, D. (1999). Grants management skills keep funded projects on target. *Nursing Economics, 17,* 131–41.

Kollock, P., & Smith, M. A. (1999). Communities in cyberspace. In M. A. Smith & K. Peter (eds.), *Communities in cyberspace* (pp. 3–27). London: Routledge.

Lakeman, R. (1997). Using the Internet for data collection in nursing research. *Computers in Nursing, 15,* 269–275.

Lindquist, R. D., Tracy, M. F., & Treat-Jacobson, D. (1995). Peer review of nursing research proposals. *American Journal of Critical Care, 4,* 59–65.

McCormick, K. A., Cohen, E., Reed, M., Sparks, S., & Wasem, C. (1996). Funding nursing informatics activities. Internet access to announcements of government funding. *Computers in Nursing, 14,* 315–322.

O'Brien, J. (1999). Writing in the body: Gender (re)production in online interaction. In M. A. Smith & K. Peter (eds.). *Communities in cyberspace* (pp. 76–103). London: Routledge.

Polit, D. F., & Hungler, B. P. (1999). *Nursing research: Principles and methods.* Philadelphia: Lippincott.

Sayer, B. (1999). Writing organization and funder profiles for a grant proposal. *Nurse Author & Editor, 9*(2), 7–9.

Turner, S. O. (1999). How to write a winning proposal. *American Journal of Nursing, 96*(7), 64–65.

U.S. Department of Health and Human Services. (2001). *Standards for privacy of individually identifiable health information—The HIPAA privacy rule.* Retrieved September 24, 2001, from http://www.hhs.gov/ocr/hipaa

Chapter 12

Institutional Review Board Issues in Internet-Based Research

Eun-Ok Im and Wonshik Chee

With recent advances in computer technologies, the Internet has become one of the fastest-growing areas in the social and behavioral sciences, and a variety of research projects are being conducted on the Internet (Jones, 1994). The Internet has also opened up a wide range of new nursing research methodologies. When searched via MEDLINE using the terms Internet, research, and nursing, 268 articles published during the period of 1960–2003 (33 years) were retrieved. All the articles were published after 1990. During the past year, 61 articles related to Internet and nursing were published. These numbers reflect the increasing number of Internet studies in the past decade.

With the increasing number of Internet studies, researchers are encountering conflicts between the risks involved in the research and the benefits of the research. Consequently, several ethical issues related to Internet research are frequently reported, and researchers have begun to discuss those issues in the literature (Buchanan, 2000; Lemmens & Elliot, 1999; Rosenoer, Isaacs, Macklin, & Silverman, 1995; Shephard, 2002). The report on the impact that the Internet has had on mental health care services and research by the National Institute of Mental Health (NIMH) is a good example of researchers' increasing concerns and discussions on the issues (NIMH, 2001).

The many disciplines already engaged in human subject research have established ethics statements to guide researchers. In the U.S., these ethical guidelines are characteristically administered through the Institutional Review Boards (IRB), and are used to guide research. Ethical issues in Internet research can be viewed within these currently available ethical guidelines provided by the IRB. However, because interrelationships between researchers and subjects in Internet research are different from those in traditional research (e.g., pen-and-pencil questionnaire, telephone survey), IRB guidelines sometimes do not fit Internet research. In this chapter, a historical review of general protections for human subjects is presented. Second, characteristics of Internet research are described. Then, according to the principles of beneficence, respect, and justice of the Belmont report, IRB issues in Internet research are discussed. Finally, suggestions for the IRB application for Internet research are included.

PROTECTION OF HUMAN SUBJECTS IN RESEARCH: A HISTORICAL REVIEW

The Nazi medical experiments of the 1930s and 1940s are the most famous example of disregard for protection of human subjects (Katz, 1996; Levine, 1986; Nuremberg Code, 1986; Steinfels & Levine, 1976). The Nazi program of research involved the use of the prisoners of war and racial "enemies" in numerous experiments designed to test the limits of human endurance and human reaction to diseases and untested drugs. They also practiced euthanasia, which involved killing various groups of people whom they considered racially impure, such as the insane, deformed, or senile. Some recent examples of unethical studies have occurred in the United States. For 40 years from 1932 to 1972, a study known as the Tuskegee Syphilis Study, sponsored by the U.S. Public Health Service, investigated the effects of syphilis among 400 men from a poor black community (Coughlin, Etheredge, Metayer, & Martin, 1996; Freimuth et al., 2001; Brandt, 1978; Rothman, 1982). Many of the subjects who consented to participate in the study were not informed about the purpose and procedures of the research, and some of them were unaware that they were subjects in a study. Medical treatment was deliberately withheld to study the course of the untreated disease even when penicillin was determined to be an effective treatment for the disease in the 1940s (Levine, 1986). In 1960, another highly publicized case of unethical research involved the injection of live cancer cells into elderly patients at the Jewish Chronic Disease Hospital in Brooklyn, without the consent of those patients (Hershey

& Miller, 1976; Levine, 1986). The patients were not informed that they were taking part in research and that the injections they received were liver cancer cells. Many other examples of studies with ethical transgressions have emerged to give ethical concerns the high visibility they have today (Polit & Hungler, 1999).

During the past four decades, largely in response to the human rights violations, various codes of ethics have been developed. One of the first internationally recognized efforts to establish ethical standards is referred to as the Nuremberg Code, developed after the Nazi atrocities were made public in the Nuremberg trials (Katz, 1996; Nuremberg Code, 1986). Several other international standards have subsequently been developed, the most notable of which is the Declaration of Helsinki, which was adopted in 1964 by the World Medical Assembly and then later revised in 1975 (Declaration of Helsinki, 1986).

In 1978, the National Commission adopted an important code of ethics for the Protection of Human Subjects of Biomedical and Behavioral Research. The commission, established by the National Research Act (Public Law 93–348), issued a report in 1978 that served as the basis for regulations affecting research sponsored by the federal government. The report, sometimes referred to as the Belmont Report, also served as a model for many of the guidelines adopted by specific disciplines. The Belmont Report, which is the basis for most IRB guidelines, articulated three primary ethical principles on which standards of ethical conduct in research are based: beneficence, respect for human dignity, and justice. The principle of beneficence requires that researchers maximize benefits and minimize harms or risks associated with research. Research-related risks must be reasonable in light of expected benefits. The principle of respect for persons (autonomy) acknowledges the dignity and freedom of every person. It requires obtaining informed consent from all potential research subjects (or their legally authorized representatives). The principle of justice requires the equitable selection and recruitment and fair treatment of research subjects.

Most disciplines have established their own code of ethics. The American Nurses Association (1975; 1985; 2001) adopted the Code of Ethics for Nurses, and the International Council of Nursing (ICN) adopted the ICN Code of Ethics for Nurses (1953; 2000). Although there is considerable overlap in the basic principles articulated in these documents, each deals with problems of particular concern to their respective disciplines.

Legal and ethical issues in Internet research recently began to be discussed (Bier, Sherblom, & Gallo, 1996; Chen, Effler, & Roche, 2001; Klemm & Nolan, 1998; Libutti, 1999; Smith & Leigh, 1997). The issues include access to the Internet, ethical consideration such as informed consent, privacy, copyright, ethics, and policy statements, ethical issues related to unanticipated consequences of research, and impact of Internet information availability on future research. International, national, and institutional efforts to develop standardized guidelines for human subject protection in electronic transmission including the Health Insurance Portability and Accountability Act (HIPAA) recommendations (Frankel & Siang, 1999; U.S. Department of Health and Human Services, 2001) have also been made. Despite these efforts, standardized guidelines for human subject protection in Internet research are not currently available to deal with the ethical issues (Frankel & Siang, 1999).

CHARACTERISTICS OF INTERNET RESEARCH

Compared with traditional research, Internet research has its own unique characteristics. These unique characteristics influence the relationships between researchers and research participants, and subsequently raise several ethical issues that have not been adequately incorporated into the currently available IRB guidelines. In this section, characteristics of Internet research are discussed under seven major categories: (a) non-face-to-face interactions, (b) real world versus fantasy world, (c) private versus public domains, (d) a selected group of research subjects, (e) prompt and better communication channels, (f) financial cost saving, and (g) unpredictability in security.

Non-Face-to-Face Interactions

One prominent characteristic of Internet research is that it is based on non-face-to-face interactions. Because of this characteristic, many ethical issues can be raised. Since researchers cannot see the participants in person, it is difficult to check if the research participants are the real persons whom they claim to be. Since people cannot see each other and online interaction strips away physical markers, researchers frequently assume that social categories based on physical characteristics would be absent and that markers such as race, gender, status, and age would be irrelevant. However, some researchers posit that the connection between racial identity and gender, and the physical body is so strong that it is simply taken for granted even in Internet interactions (Burkhalter, 1999). In online interactions, racial identity springs from participants' perspectives on racial issues rather than from physical cues, and the reliance on a participant's written words as a source of racial identity also reverses the usual sequence in stereotyping.

Another interesting recent finding on Internet interactions is that gender is reintroduced in Internet interactions in a more limited and stereotyped manner than exists in embodied interaction (O'Brien, 1999). Since there are no limitations to how one might describe oneself in cyberspace, people recreate themselves as stereotypical ideals, and this "hyper-gendering" is especially prevalent among those who attempt to cross-dress (i.e. males presenting themselves as females).

Real World Versus Fantasy World

As O'Brien (1999) pointed out, there is also strain between those who view online interactions as an opportunity to perform a variety of perhaps fabricated roles versus those who see cyberspace as a new communication medium between real people. The most difficult issue to deal with in Internet research would be how to establish ways of underscoring real versus fictitious sites so that researchers can reliably distinguish real authenticity from authentic fantasy. On the Internet, because of non-face-to-face interactions, it is difficult to differentiate whether this is a site having more to do with theater versus a site where identity is tied in some reliable way to one's real-world embodied self. The issue of real authenticity and authentic fantasy is sometimes problematic because research assumes authentic interactions between researchers and research participants.

Public Versus Private Domains

The realities of computer technology make it possible for researchers to turn the Internet into a realm where activities and habits are monitored and recorded without potential research participants' knowledge or consent. The Internet interactions and activities can be private or public depending on the characteristics of the interactions and how members of the Internet communities/groups perceive the interactions. There has been much debate regarding whether the Internet is in a private or public realm (Mann & Stewart, 2000). Correll (1995) conducted an ethnographic study through a lesbian cyber café, and found that the creation and maintenance of physical space is one of the key rituals in the organization of interaction. In a space where setting can only be evoked textually, patrons of the cyber café used descriptions of physical artifacts to organize the spaces of interaction, to define relationships to each other, and to create and maintain a social order. This kind of reference to town halls, town pumps, villages, and cafes all give ample testimony to an overriding definition of online forums as public status. These virtual spaces are communal spaces, and this implies that the interaction which occurs within them is also public and thus falls within the remit of an observational sociology which is directed at understanding behavior in public spaces whether on or off-line (Correll, 1995).

In general, however, if data on identifiable private information are obtained and/or if its members consider it private (researchers may find this information from its owner or moderator), the Internet actions should be regarded as private communication that is not allowed to be interrupted or observed. Private information usually refers to information about behavior that occurs in contexts in which an individual can reasonably expect that no observation or recording is taking place. Private information also refers to information which has been provided for specific purposes by an individual and which the individual can reasonably expect not to be disclosed in public (Correll, 1995). Therefore, if members of the Internet communities/groups perceive them as private, researchers should go through appropriate channels to obtain consent, permission, and guidelines for his/her participation or observation of the Internet communities/groups.

A Selected Group of Research Subjects

The most recent survey by Georgia Tech Graphics Visualization and Usability Center (1999) indicated that Internet users tend to be a select sample of well-educated, literate, and articulate people who are skilled users of computers and have access to the Internet. According to the tenth survey by the Georgia Tech Graphics Visualization and Usability Center (Lacroiz, Backus, & Lyon, 1994) on the Internet use, 33% of the participants were female, and the percentage decreased compared with previous surveys. Participants tended to be highly educated with 87.8% having at least some college experience and 59.3% having obtained at least one degree. The average age of the survey participants was 37.6 years old and participants were predominantly white (87.2%). Younger participants were more diverse racially than older participants. Among participants who had been online for less than a year, 3.8% were African-American. About 47.6% were married and 31.7% were single. Many Internet users work in university education (11.6%), information services (6.8%), and software (6.0%). Average household income of the Internet users was $57,300 (U. S.). From the survey findings, we can say that Internet users frequently do not represent research populations that are targeted for nursing research. Especially when studying patients with critical conditions such as cancer survivors, respondents tend to be healthy persons because they have to be able to express their experiences by typing into a computer and using an electronic method of communication (Fawcett & Buhle, 1995; Senior & Smith, 1999). Therefore, limitations in generalizability are frequently pointed out as one of the major weaknesses of Internet research.

Prompt and Better Communication Channels

The Internet provides a more immediate and prompt channel for communication between researchers and research participants. Lakeman (1997) reported that people responded more promptly with e-mail, and that differences in time zones and geographic distance were not important issues in using the Internet. Research participants can also more easily ask questions and get answers by e-mail. Murray (1995) also described how in his research using e-mail, after starting interviews with structured questions, the interviews became progressively unstructured and varied in content depending on the interviewee's interests. Im and Chee (2001) asserted that, compared with traditional data collection methods, data collection through the Internet and e-mail may provide better opportunities for research participants to get informed. Another unique feature of Internet communication is that the Internet allows both asynchronous and synchronous interactions (Lakeman, 1998). Asynchronous interaction allows people on very different schedules or in distant time zones to exchange messages and sustain discussions. Synchronous interaction allows a group of people to communicate simultaneously, directly, and without time delay.

Financial Cost Saving

Financial cost savings are possible with Internet research because long distance travel, paper, pencils, photocopying, and mailing are not required

(Frandsen, 1997; Lakeman, 1998). Therefore, researchers who plan to use the Internet as a data collection method usually expect a lower cost compared with traditional data collection methods. However, Im and Chee (2001) found that, instead of paper, pencil, photocopying, and mailing costs, Internet research required a computer server, a printer, computer software, and consumable computer supplies (e.g., floppy diskettes, printer cartridges). Subsequently, the cost may be much more expensive compared with traditional survey methods.

Unpredictability in Security

Although advances in computer technologies have made tremendous strides in terms of Internet security, there is still no completely secure interaction online (Im & Chee, 2001; Kelly & McKenzie, 2002). E-mail can be intercepted and channels of delivery are not direct and "pure." Intrusion by outsiders can happen at any time. Sometimes, Internet users are not aware that they are monitored and data about them are collected (e.g., via "cookies" on a website). For example, registration with a website can enable the website to keep track of what Internet users view or spend online, and the information may be passed on to third parties. Therefore, unpredictability in security is an important consideration when conducting Internet research.

IRB ISSUES IN INTERNET RESEARCH

Because of the nature of Internet interactions, there exist several ethical issues in Internet research. In the following section, IRB issues are discussed as related to the three principles of the Belmont report: beneficence, respect, and justice.

Beneficence

The principle of beneficence obligates researchers to balance potential benefits and risks of research. Thus, researchers should maximize possible benefits from the research and minimize harms and risks to their subjects. Benefits mean gains to society or science through contribution to the knowledge base, gains to the individual through improved well-being, or empowerment of the individual by giving him or her a voice

(Frankel & Siang, 1999). Harms may refer to death and injury, psychological abuse, loss of privacy and public exposure, and may not only affect individuals but specific subgroups as well (Frankel & Siang, 1999).

Usually, even in Internet research, benefits to research participants tend to be limited to the ability to collect useful data and extend knowledge on a specific area of research interest. In Internet research, the risk of death is minimal. However, questions on sampling techniques and the validity and reliability of the data collected can be raised. Researchers could reach potential research participants residing in dispersed areas, and the Internet could provide national and international communication channels. However, at the same time, because Internet interactions are non-face-to-face, the Internet can easily mislead researchers about research participants' geographical location, gender, or race (Murray & Sixsmith, 1998). Furthermore, as discussed above, individuals who respond to Internet-based research tend to be a select population, which means that a sample can be skewed in terms of gender, race, and geographical distribution. Therefore, limitations in generalizability can be of significant concern in Internet research. This concern can be detrimental to potential results that researchers claim. In other words, Internet research can result in misleading findings and possibly misguide policy if policy makers rely upon the data.

In Internet research, research subjects are less likely to experience physical injury as may happen with other types of traditional research conducted in the physical world (Frankel & Siang, 1999). Most risks/harms by Internet research can be grouped as minimal psychological discomforts, but this does not mean that researchers can be less vigilant of Internet research. As frequently noted in recent news and media, Internet interactions can be susceptible to hacking and intrusion by outsiders, and no system is 100% safe. Furthermore, lack of knowledge on technical and storage capabilities of Internet technologies can possibly elevate the risk. For example, participants may not know that there is a record of the exchange in a cache somewhere on their system or saved in their Internet service provider's server's log files (Murray & Sixsmith, 1998). Participants may also not know that outdated or poorly designed security measures used in old computers may create more opportunity for risky exposure.

Another potential risk involved in Internet research would be loss of privacy. Studies have reported that people tend to become more open online than they are in person (Childress & Asamen, 1998; Reid, 1996). With a false expectation of privacy, people tend to reveal more than what they usually do in the physical world. This tendency sometimes results in a vulnerability to privacy invasions by outsiders. Indeed, negative experiences related to privacy invasions by outsiders have been frequently reported in the literature (Finn & Lavitt, 1994; King, 1996).

Respect

The principle of respect requires that subjects be treated with respect as autonomous agents and affirms that those persons with diminished autonomy are entitled to special protection. This principle is reflected in the process of informed consent in the IRB, through which the risks and benefits of the research are fully disclosed to the research subjects. Because of differences in communication characteristics between Internet interactions and interpersonal relationships in the physical world, there are several IRB issues in terms of the principle of respect in Internet research. First of all, the issues related to private versus public domains are raised in terms of when informed consent should be obtained. If participants of the specific Internet communities/groups perceive that their online communities/groups are private, researchers should obtain consent for data collection. On the contrary, if participants perceive that their communities/groups are public, researchers may be exempt from obtaining consent for data collected from the public domain. In traditional research, we can clearly determine which is in the public domain. For example, we can clearly see that data collected from television, public records, radio, printed books, conferences, or in public spaces such as parks belong to the public domain. However, determining if an online community/group is in the public domain is not simple. In most cases, cyberspace such as newsgroups, listservs, Internet Relay Chats (IRCs), and Multi-User Dungeons (MUDs) can be clearly viewed as part of the public domain because these are accessible to anyone. However, some of them that are not open to the public are certainly in the private domain.

The next issue in terms of the informed consent is how to obtain it. In traditional research conducted in the physical world, researchers can obtain informed consent through written or verbal consent to participate in the study. In Internet research, usually, researchers ask the subjects to click "I agree to participate" to obtain informed consent. In a sense, research participants can more easily ask questions and get answers through the Internet interactions compared with traditional quantitative research methods including self-administered questionnaires (Im & Chee, 2001; Lakeman, 1997). In this regard, Internet research may provide better opportunities for research participants to get informed about the research and self-determine their participation. However, informed consent in Internet research is still problematic because it is difficult to ensure that the research subjects who agree to participate are the real persons who meet the inclusion criteria. While research assumes authentic interactions between researchers and research participants, it is questionable how authentic the interactions and the phenomena reported and/or explored through the Internet can be in reality (Frankel & Siang, 1999). Furthermore, in Internet research, full disclosure is impossible in most cases because researchers cannot guarantee or fully disclose potential risks and benefits. There are no systems that are 100% safe and hacking-free.

Another IRB issue would be potential violation of voluntariness. "Error messages" are frequently used in commercial Internet surveys and/or questionnaires. Whenever a participant skips a question, an error message (reminding the participant that he/she has not answered the specific question) usually appears on the screen, and a computer server-side program does not process the questionnaire until the participant answers the missed question. To minimize errors in data entry by the participants, researchers frequently plan to use error messages as in commercial Internet surveys and/or questionnaires. However, in research studies among human subjects, researchers should allow the participants to refuse to answer any questions that they feel uncomfortable about and to withdraw their participation when they want. Therefore, "error messages" that do not allow the participants to skip the questions that they do not want to answer are violating "voluntariness" of participation.

Justice

The principle of justice seeks a fair distribution of the burdens and benefits associated with research so that certain individuals or groups do not bear disproportionate risks while others reap the benefits. An injustice occurs when certain persons are denied benefits that are rightfully due to them or when burdens are not distributed fairly (Beauchamp & Childress, 1994). This means that selection and recruitment of participants should occur while ensuring that subjects are selected for reasons directly related to the problem being studied instead of for their easy availability, compromised position, or tractability. In Internet research, as mentioned above, participants tend to be a select group who tend to be in high-income brackets, highly educated, and white males. Therefore, in a sense, Internet research violates this principle by nature. Furthermore, under the circumstances that subjects' real identities are just assumed to be authentic, this principle of justice may not be easily ensured in Internet research. In traditional research, researchers need to consider mediating factors including gender, race, age, and socioeconomic status in the selection of their subjects and try to maximize the generalizability of study results. In Internet research, this will be one of the most difficult tasks to conduct because of the nature of Internet interactions and characteristics of current Internet users. Because researchers cannot guarantee the real identity of the research participants (and cannot determine sociodemographic characteristics of the participants), controlling specific factors is virtually impossible.

SUGGESTIONS FOR PREPARATION OF IRB PROTOCOLS FOR INTERNET RESEARCH

In this chapter, a historical review of protection of human subjects in research in general is provided. Then, characteristics of Internet research and IRB issues in Internet research are discussed. As discussed in the sections on characteristics of Internet research and IRB issues in Internet research, Internet research is different from traditional research by nature. Because of its select groups of subjects, non-face-to-face interactions, difficulties in ensuring authenticity of interactions, and vague distinctions of private and public domains on the Internet, Internet research may violate the principles of beneficence, respect, and justice in part. Therefore, when preparing the IRB protocol, researchers need to give special attention to the potential IRB issues. Based on the above discussions on the IRB issues, the following suggestions are made for researchers who are considering using the Internet as a data collection method or medium.

First, researchers need to identify aspects of existing ethical guidelines and policies that can be applied to Internet research (e.g., HIPAA regulations, SANS/FBI suggestions, the Association of Internet Researchers (AoIR)'s Internet research ethics, etc.). At the same time, researchers need to identify how their institutions' IRBs currently handle ethical issues in Internet research. With the increasing number of Internet studies, many institutions have begun to develop their own policies and regulations related to Internet research (e.g., University of Illinois, New York University, University of Wisconsin). In addition, researchers need to check ethical guidelines by their professional organizations (e.g., ANA's ethical guidelines).

Second, researchers need to clarify if the Internet communities/groups that researchers are going to explore are in private and/or public domains. The most efficient and clear way to determine if the Internet communities/groups are in private or public domains would be a direct contact to the community/group owners and/or webmasters. Alternatively, researchers can contact and ask all members of the community/group what they perceive the status to be. Researchers may also contact the communities to have consultation in planning research and interpreting results regarding the communities' own perceived benefits and harms, their expectations of privacy, and the information that the potential participants believe they should know before giving consent to participate in the research.

Third, as in traditional research, researchers need to be specific about the possible benefits and harms to their subjects, how they will minimize risks, and how they will secure informed consent from prospective subjects. Because of the technical nature of Internet research, researchers need to consult with their institutions' technology system administrators regarding the technical aspects of their research, and understand the strengths and limitations of the research medium. Through this process researchers can become more informed about potential benefits and harms/risks involved in the technologies they plan to use.

Fourth, researchers need to understand potential vulnerabilities of research subjects with respect to Internet research and make it clear in the research proposal how they will protect vulnerable research subjects. Especially, when researchers involve international participants through the Internet, researchers need to consider what would be potential unfair conditions for them (e.g., language, timing, access to the Internet), and be sensitive to cultural or political factors that affect the vulnerability of those participants.

Finally, researchers need to make it clear in the informed consent that full disclosure is impossible in the Internet interactions because no systems are 100% safe and hacking-proof. Potential research participants need to understand potential technical difficulties in the security of Internet interactions because of daily changes in Internet technologies. At the same time, researchers need to understand the needs for regular updates of computer systems and the software that they are using for the Internet research, and regularly update whenever new versions or new security measures are available.

REFERENCES

American Nurses Association (ANA). (1975). *Human rights guidelines for nurses in clinical and other research.* Kansas City, MO: Author.

American Nurses Association (ANA). (1985). *Human rights guidelines for nurses in clinical and other research.* Kansas City, MO: Author.

American Nurses Association (ANA). (2001). *Human rights guidelines for nurses in clinical and other research.* Kansas City, MO: Author.

Beauchamp, T., & Childress, J. (1994). *Principles of biomedical ethics* (4th ed.). Oxford, England: Oxford University Press.

Bier, M.C., Sherblom, S.A., & Gallo, M.A., (1996). Ethical issues in a study of Internet use: Uncertainty, responsibility, and the spirit of research relationships. *Ethics and Behavior, 6,*141–51.

Brandt, A. M. (1978). Racism and research: The case of the Tuskegee Syphilis Study. *Hastings Center Report, 8,* 21–29

Buchanan, E. A. (2000). Ethics, qualitative research, and ethnography in virtual space. *Journal of Information Ethics, 9,* 82–87.

Burkhalter, B. (1999). Reading race online: Discovering racial identity in Usenet discussions. In M. A. Smith & K. Peter (Eds.), *Communities in cyberspace* (pp. 60–75). London & New York: Routledge.

Chen, S.L., Effler, J.R., & Roche, A.L. (2001). Using Internet services to generate a research sampling frame. *Nursing Health Science, 3,* 15–18.

Childress, C. A., & Asamen, J. K. (1998). The emerging relationship of psychology and the Internet: Proposed guidelines for conducting research. *Ethics and Behavior, 8*(1), 19–35.

Correll, S. (1995). The ethnography of an electronic bar: The lesbian café. *Journal of Contemporary Ethnography, 24,* 270–298.

Coughlin, S. S., Etheredge, G. D., Metayer, C., & Martin, S. A., Jr. (1996). Remember Tuskegee: Public health student knowledge of the ethical significance of the Tuskegee Syphilis Study. *American Journal of Preventive Medicine, 12,* 242–246

Declaration of Helsinki. (1986). In R. J. Levine (Ed.), *Ethics and regulations of clinical research* (2nd ed., pp. 427–429). Baltimore: Urban & Schwarzenberg.

Fawcett, J. F., & Buhle, E. L. (1995). Using the Internet for data collection. *Computers in Nursing, 13,* 273–279.

Finn, J., & Lavitt, M. (1994). Computer based self-help group for sexual abuse survivors. *Social Work with Groups, 17,* 21–46.

Frandsen, J. L. (1997). The use of computers in cancer pain management. *Seminars in Oncology Nursing, 13,* 49–56.

Frankel, M. S., & Siang, S. (1999). Ethical and legal aspects of human subjects research on the Internet. Retrieved April 17, 2003, from http://www.aaas.org/spp/dspp/sfrl/projects/intres/main.htm.

Freimuth, V. S., Quinn, S. C., Thomas, S. B., Cole, G., Zook, E, & Duncan, T. (2001). African Americans' views on research and the Tuskegee Syphilis Study. *Social Science Medicine, 52,* 797–808.

Georgia Tech Graphics Visualization and Usability Centre. (1999). *GVU's 10th WWW user survey* [online]. Available at: http://www.gvu.gatech.edu/user_surveys/survey_1998_10/ tenthreport.html

Hershey, N., & Miller, R. D. (1976). *Human experimentation and the law.* Germantown, MD: Aspen.

Im, E. O., & Chee, W. (2001). A feminist critique on the use of the Internet in nursing research. *Advances in Nursing Science, 23*(4), 67–82.

International Council of Nursing (ICN). (1953). *Code of ethics.* Geneva, Switzerland: The Author.

International Council of Nursing (ICN). (2000). *Code of ethics.* Geneva, Switzerland: The Author.

Jones, R. A. (1994). The ethics of research in cyberspace. *Internet Research, 4,* 30–35.

Katz, J. (1996). The Nuremberg Code and the Nuremberg Trial: A reappraisal. *Journal of the American Medical Association, 276*(20), 1662–1666.

Kelly, G., & McKenzie, B. (2002). Security, privacy, and confidentiality issues on the Internet. *Journal of Medical Internet Research, 4*(2), e12.

King, S. A. (1996). Researching Internet communities: Proposed ethical guidelines for the reporting of results. *The Information Society, 12,* 119–127.

Klemm, P., & Nolan, M.T. (1998). Internet cancer support groups: Legal and ethical issues for nurse researchers. *Oncology Nursing Forum, 25,* 673–6.

Lacroiz, E. M., Backus, J. E., & Lyon, B. J. (1994). Service providers and users discover the Internet. *Bulletin of the Medical Library Association, 82,* 412–418.

Lakeman, R. (1997). Using the Internet for data collection in nursing research. *Computers in Nursing, 15,* 269–275.

Lakeman, R. (1998). The Internet: Facilitating an international nursing culture for psychiatric nurses. *Computers in Nursing, 16,* 87–89.

Lemmens, T., & Elliot, C. (1999). Guinea pigs on the payroll: The ethics of paying research subjects. *Accounting Research Journal, 7,* 3–20.

Levine, R. J. (1986). *Ethics and regulation of clinical research* (2nd ed.). Baltimore & Munich, Germany: Urban & Schwarzenberg.

Libutti, P.O., (1999). The Internet and qualitative research: Opportunities and constraints on analysis of cyberspace discourse. In M. Kopala & L. A. Suzuki,(Eds.). *Using qualitative methods in psychology* (pp. 77-88). Thousand Oaks, CA: Sage.

Mann, C., & Stewart, F. (2000). *Internet communication and qualitative research: A handbook for researching online.* Thousand Oaks, CA: Sage.

Murray, C. D., & Sixsmith, J. (1998). E-mail: A qualitative research medium for interviewing? *International Journal of Social Research Methodology, 1,* 103–121.

Murray, P. J. (1995). Using the Internet for gathering data and conducting research: Faster than the mail, cheaper than the phone. *Computers in Nursing, 13,* 206–209.

National Commission for the Protection of Human Subjects of Biomedical and Behavioral Research. (1978). *Belmont report: Ethical principles and guidelines for research involving human subjects.* (DHEW Publication No. (05) 78–0012.) Washington, DC: U.S. Government Printing Office.

National Institute of Mental Health (NIMH). (2001). *Internet ethics workshop—"Consider this" Cyber interventions in mental health-ethical considerations.* Bethesda, MD: NIMH Publications.

Nuremberg Code. (1986). In R. J. Levine (Ed.), *Ethics and regulation of clinical research* (2nd ed., pp. 425–426). Baltimore & Munich, Germany: Urban & Schwarzenberg.

O'Brien, J. (1999). Writing in the body: Gender (re)production in online interaction. In M. A. Smith & K. Peter (Eds.), *Communities in cyberspace* (pp. 76–105). London & New York: Routledge.

Polit, D., & Hungler, B. P. (1999). *Nursing research: Principles and methods (6th ed.).* Philadelphia: Lippincott.

Reid, E. (1996). Informed consent in the study of online communities: A reflection on the effects of computer-mediated social research. *The Information Society, 12,* 169–174.

Rosenoer, J., Isaacs, S., Macklin, R., & Silverman, S. (1995). Observational research on the electronic superhighway; Problems on the Internet: A lawyer's perspective; The networker's perspective; Bioethics perspective; User's perspective. *Ethics Behavior, 5,* 105–118.

Rothman, D. J. (1982). Were Tuskegee & Willowbrook 'studies in nature'? *Hastings Center Report, 12,* 5–7.

Senior, C., & Smith, M. (1999). The Internet . . . A possible research tool? *Psychologist, 12,* 442–444.

Shephard, R. J. (2002). Ethics in exercise science research. *Sports Medicine, 32,* 169–183.

Smith, M. A., & Leigh, B. (1997). Virtual subjects: Using the Internet as an alternative source of subjects and research environment. *Behavior Research Methods, Instruments, and Computers, 29,* 496–505.

Steinfels, P., & Levine, C. (1976). Biomedical ethics and the shadow of Nazism. *Hastings Center Report, 6,* 1–20.

U.S. Department of Health and Human Services. (2001). *Standards for privacy of individually identifiable health information—The HIPAA privacy rule.* Retrieved September 24, 2001, from http://www.hhs.gov/ocr/hipaa

Chapter 13

Hardware and Software Options

John M. Clochesy

T he Internet provides numerous opportunities for nurses conducting research. Identifying how information technologies can contribute to research and selecting the most appropriate software and hardware can be a daunting task. This chapter provides information on questions to ask and decisions to consider to optimize Internet use in nursing research.

SPECIFYING THE NEEDS

Specifying "what needs to be done" is the first step in using various information technologies in research. Investigators need to consider a wide range of factors, including: tasks to be accomplished, requirements for interoperability and compatibility, location where various research activities must or preferentially should occur, desirability of mobile use of technology, desirability of precise location or distance measures (geospatial data), usefulness of real-time video capture, data visualization, including three- and four-dimensional options, and the quantity of data to be stored.

Identifying Software

Once project specifications have been completed, the software necessary to accomplish them can be identified. Decisions about software

are best made before "hardware" or devices are selected since some crucial or preferred software may not be available for particular operating systems or hardware configurations. Software categories that should be considered include data acquisition (for biophysical data), data capture (for observational and survey data), database, graphics, and statistical analysis.

Data acquisition and capture. Data acquisition of biophysical data involves the use of "firmware" (computer cards) and associated software. These software-hardware combinations are especially useful with sensors that measure variables frequently, as often as several hundred times per second if necessary. The total number of discrete measurements that can be recorded is limited primarily by the data storage space available. Major vendors of data acquisition solutions used in health science research include Gould Instrument Systems (Valley View, OH) at: http://www.gouldis.com, Keithley Instruments (Cleveland, OH) at: http://www.keithley.com, and National Instruments (Austin, TX) at: http://www.ni.com.

Historically, data capture of observations or survey responses were performed with paper and pencil. Software facilitates data entry and minimizes cost of data capture. Software may allow direct entry into a personal digital assistant or laptop computer or the scanning of forms marked by observers and/or informants. Popular software solutions include SNAP Survey Software 7 (Mercator Research Group, Bristol UK) at: http://www.mercatorresearch.com and TELEform 8.2 (Cardiff Software, Vista, CA) at: http://www.cardiff.com/TELEform/.

Database systems. Database systems are the foundation of data management processes. Databases can be relational, "flat" file, object-oriented, XML, or geospatial in nature.

Relational databases. The most frequently used relational databases are those that must manage its stored data using only its relational capabilities relational databases are compliant with open database connectivity (ODBC) and structured query language (SQL) standards. These standards are important since they assure the ability to link other programs to enter data, to manipulate data, and to retrieve data and send it to the software of choice to perform data visualization and statistical analysis.

Software for large relational databases include Oracle (Redwood Shores, CA) at: http://www.oracle.com, Sybase (Dublin, CA) at: http://www.sybase.com, DB2 (IBM, White Plains, NY) at: http://www-3.ibm.com/software/data/db2/, and SQL Server (Microsoft, Redmond,

WA) at: http://www.microsoft.com. Oracle is available for most platforms. It is widely used on Windows and Linux systems. Sybase is available for Windows and various forms of Unix (Solaris, Linux, AIX, HP UX).

Smaller projects more commonly use MS Access and Visual FoxPro (Microsoft), Corel Paradox (Ottawa, Ontario) at: http:// www.corel.com, or MySQL at: http://www.mysql.com. MS Access, Visual FoxPro and Paradox are all available for Windows. MySQL is available for many platforms including Windows and most versions of Unix including Mac OS X and SGI IRIX. A relative newcomer to relational database software is the open source Firebird 1.5 at: http://firebird.sourceforge.net. This database system is available for Windows, Linux and other Unix platforms.

Flat file databases. A relatively simple database system in which each database is contained in a single table. The most common "flat" file databases used in nursing research are MS Excel (Microsoft) and SPSS (Chicago, IL) at: http://www.spss.com. These databases are based on spreadsheets of rows and columns of numbers. For small studies of limited complexity, this type of file may be sufficient. Excel is available for Windows and Mac OS X. A version is available for Pocket PC-based personal digital assistants.

Other databases. Nurses are just beginning to use newer database technologies. These technologies include object-oriented databases, XML databases, and geographic information system (GIS) databases. XML database is a collection of data that is located in a database management system. GIS is a database that includes geographic data and organizes it in a way that is useful. Object-oriented database are ones that use object programming language. Of these newer technologies, geospatial databases (geographic information systems) may serve a unique role in community health, epidemiologic, and public policy research. A major vendor of GIS software, data, and maps is ESRI (Redlands, CA) at: http://www.esri.com. The selection of any database is based on data type and need for manipulation, user expertise, and level of support available to the research team.

Compatible platforms. "Platforms" refers to the operating system (and, at times, the central processing unit or CPU of the computer) upon which application software runs. Software that has instructions "compiled" for one operating system and CPU will not operate properly on other operating systems or computers. If several types of devices will be used in a project, such as personal digital assistants, laptop computers, and workstations or servers, it is important to identify at the outset if each of these devices will be required to run the same or compatible software.

One of the most widely-used platforms is the Windows family of operating systems from Microsoft that are designed for 32-bit CPUs such as those from Advanced Micro Devices (Sunnyvale, CA) at: http://www.amd.com and Intel (Santa Clara, CA) at: http://www.intel.com. Selecting Windows as the operating system may be preferable if you plan on using a range of devices. Compatible operating systems from the Windows family include Pocket PC 2003, Windows XP, and Windows XP Professional Tablet PC Edition.

Mac OS X (Apple Computer, Cupertino, CA) at: http://www.apple.com is built upon BSD Unix (Berkley Software Design), a very stable operating system used to power many high-end workstations and servers. The Apple G5 computers are based on a powerful 64-bit processor from IBM. The combination of Mac OS X and the G5 is an ideal, cost-effective choice for computer-intensive applications where the desired software is available.

Linux and other Unix "flavors" are popular in data centers. Many high-end workstations and servers are based on Linux or other versions of Unix. This is a very stable operating system. It is often the least expensive to implement and maintain in the data server and Web server environment. Linux is now found on a few personal digital assistants (PDAs).

The Palm OS (Palm Source) is found on PDAs from Palm (Handspring, Palm), Sony (Clie), and Symbol. Smartphones based on the Palm OS are available from Samsung.

Selecting Hardware

Nurse researchers using the Internet will make several "hardware" or equipment choices. Final equipment selection is based on software and operating system compatibility with desired hardware as well as many straightforward factors such as cost, ease of use, and durability.

"Large" systems. It is useful to discuss any "large" system decisions with the information technology support staff available. The technologies found in desktop computers, workstations, and servers are changing rapidly. Most researchers do not have large enough projects to justify dedicated workstations or servers. It may be prudent to explore use of existing computing resources at the university, hospital, or clinic for data storage and warehousing.

Mobile systems. Compatibility, connectivity, and expandability are key factors when choosing from among the ever-growing selection of mobile devices. Compatibility issues are operating system and software. If mobile devices must be compatible with desktops, a workstation or server care is needed to ensure compatibility.

Connectivity relates to the type and number of "ports" or connectors available on the device. The types of ports that may be desirable include universal serial bus (USB), FireWire (also called iLink or IEEE 1394), and video graphics array (VGA). The USB and firewire ports allow additional devices and disk drives to be attached. At a minimum, a USB port version 1.1 should be present. USB 2.0 ports communicate at much faster speeds. Firewire ports are especially useful if you are making digital video recordings. Add-in memory cards may be useful and come in several formats and storage capacities. The most commonly used memory card is Compact Flash (CF). Other popular formats are Sony's Memory Stick and Memory Stick Pro, Secure Digital (SD), Smart Media, and xD Card. Many of the card formats come in capacities up to 1 GB.

Laptop computers. Laptop computers have most of the functionality of larger "desktop" systems. Laptop computers should be considered when a mobile workstation is desired. Laptop computers have full-size keyboards that facilitate data entry. Most laptop computers weigh 4 to 7 or 8 pounds.

Sub-notebook. Sub-notebook computers lack optical disk drives such as CD and DVD drives. They are smaller and lighter than notebook computers, often about 2 pounds. While these devices are great for giving presentations while traveling and taking notes in meetings, the smaller keyboard and video display are a drawback for general use.

Personal digital assistants. Personal digital assistants are very popular. They are the outgrowth of electronic personal organizers (phone books with calendars). Generally small, PDAs often weigh a mere 5 to 8 ounces. PDAs can be useful in collecting real-time observational data. Due to the small size and ubiquity, they are relatively unobtrusive in public settings.

Tablet PCs. Tablet PCs combine the "pen" input of PDAs with the functionality of a laptop or sub-notebook computer. These devices may be the answer when the PDA is not powerful enough or the display is too small. Toshiba (http://www.toshiba.com) is developing a unique twist to the Tablet PC, called the "Dynasheet." It is to function like a Tablet PC with a flexible display that can be rolled up and put into a pocket or bag. This type of device will be useful for "field" research conducted by community health nurses and others.

Storage Devices

Optical disk drives. Optical drives use lasers to read and write data from plastic disks. These drives are commonly known as CD and DVD drives. The most commonly used CD drive is a CD-RW or CD-rewriteable drive. Blank CDs hold 640 or 700 MB of data. DVD-ROM is a drive that allows a computer to read DVDs with data or video files. There are several writeable DVD formats (DVD-RAM, DVD-R, DVD-RW, DVD+R, DVD+RW). The differences are technical, but can cause problems with compatibility. Recently, DVD drives that can read and write all of these formats became available. A multi-format DVD drive would facilitate data sharing while minimizing problems with incompatible disks. Recordable DVDs hold 4.7 GB of data (approximately 7.3 standard CDs).

Removable and portable disks. Iomega (San Diego, CA) at: http://www.iomega.com has long been the major supplier of removable media drives. Their ZIP drives accept removable disks that store 100 MB, 250 MB, or 750 MB each. A decline in the use of these drives has occurred with the ubiquity of CD-RW drives and the low cost of CD disks. Portable hard drives that attach to a USB or FireWire port play an ever-increasing role in data mobility and for use in back up.

Web Cams

Web-attached video cameras are widely used for videoconferencing, video recording, and monitoring geographic areas (such as traffic patterns and illegal activities by police). Web cams can be attached to a computer or PDA either directly or by cable to the device's USB port. Stand-alone cameras can be attached directly to a network by an Ethernet cable or by wireless networking (e.g. Wi-Fi, 802.11b). Some cameras have remote controls that allow researchers to reposition the camera. Some cameras have automatic or manual controls for exposure to allow for optimal use under the greatest range of lighting conditions.

GETTING CONNECTED

If nurse researchers are to use the Internet for research, they must be connected. There are several ways to connect to the Internet. Members of any given research team use many of these "ways to connect" just like individuals use a variety of modes of transportation to get to and from the workplace. From the laboratory or office, most researchers connect to the Internet through a corporate local area network (LAN). LANs can be based on fiber optic cables or twisted pairs of copper wires. Speed of LANs are described as 10 Mbps, 100 Mbps, or 1000 Mbps (or a gigabit per second). The speed of the LAN is the greatest speed with which systems attached directly to the local network can communicate with each other. The speed with which one can connect to another system outside the LAN is related to the total amount of traffic on the "commodity Internet" much like the amount of automobile traffic on a freeway at any given time. A useful tool to test the speed of your connection to the Internet is found in the "Our Tools" section at: http://www.broadbandreports.com.

Access to the "commodity Internet" is purchased from an Internet Service Provider (ISP). Access can be dial-up, broadband, or wireless. Dial-up service is sufficient when intermittent access to the Internet is required for transmitting or receiving small amounts of information. Dial-up service costs range from $9.95 per month to the $21.95 range depending on ISP and service plan. National ISPs that offer dial-up service include America Online (AOL), Earthlink and MSN. There are many local or regional ISPs as well. Before selecting an ISP, check to make certain that there are access (phone) numbers that are local calls from the locations that you need. If you need to dial a long distance number or a toll-free number (added fee), dial-up service may cost as much or more than other choices. In selecting an ISP, make certain that you can use virtual private network (VPN) software over their service if you are transmitting or accessing data, such as personal health information, that needs to be kept confidential.

When continuous access is needed and/or large amounts of data must be exchanged, broadband is preferable. The two most common broadband solutions are the service provided by digital cable companies and digital subscriber line (DSL) service provided by telephone companies. DSL can frequently be purchased from an ISP who "buys" the DSL access from the telephone company. DSL and cable broadband cost approximately $50 per month. Additional broadband solutions include wireless, fixed wireless, and satellite options.

Wireless Internet access is available through two technologies, the wireless LAN (based on Wi-Fi, 802.11 standards) and "cellular" phone systems (CDMA 1xRTT or GPRS). Wireless access is ideal where members of the team may be working in a dynamic environment, collecting and entering data in locations that change frequently. The limitations to wireless Internet access are the availability of wireless access points ("hot spots") and cellular-based Internet services. Wireless Internet access is available from many "cellular" telephone service providers. National providers include: ATT Wireless which operates two systems, GoPorts (802.11b) and PCS (GPRS) (http://www.attwireless.com). Sprint's PCS Vision is based on CDMA 1xRTTT (http:// www.sprintpcs. com). T-Mobile operates two systems, HotSpots (802.11b) and PCS (GPRS) (http://www.t-mobile.com). Verizon offers Express Network (CDMA 1xRTT) (http://www.verizonwireless.com). In some circumstances, researchers will use mobile devices that include Wi-Fi and cellular Internet access that automatically switches to whichever signal is strongest. Fixed wireless or the wireless metropolitan area network (MAN) is based on an evolving standard (IEEE 802.16). It is expected that this form of high-speed wireless Internet access will become commercially available in 2005.

While rarely used by nurse researchers, a broadband connection can be obtained from a satellite Internet service provider. Cost and interference from weather limit the number of users. This type of broadband access is usually reserved for locations where other options are not available (rural settings too far from a central switching office, for example).

MAINTAINING SECURITY

The final area that needs to be addressed when using Internet technologies for nursing research is security of data and your systems. The foundation of a security system is good virus protection software that automatically updates itself as new viruses are identified. Commonly used virus protection solutions are Symantec's Norton Anti-Virus (http://www.symantec.com) and McAfee's Virus Scan (http://www.mcafee. com). Firewalls minimize intrusion into your computer systems from others using the Internet. Firewalls can make your computer appear invisible to the Internet. Firewall software solutions for individual computers or small networks are available from Zone Laboratories, and Zone Alarm (http://www.zonealarm.com) in addition to Symantec and McAfee.

All devices should be password protected. For systems that contain personal health information of research subjects, biometric authentication, such as fingerprint, may be desirable. Biometric authentication is available as a standard feature on some laptop computers and PDAs. It can be added to many others. Finally, when communicating over wireless connections or the commodity Internet, it is advisable to establish a virtual private network (VPN) that "tunnels" through the Internet and attaches to your other systems. VPN encrypts all data transmission, protecting subjects and data integrity.

Chapter 14

Security for Research Office Computers and Databases

Mary L. McHugh

A s researchers use Internet resources, it is wise to keep in mind that a variety of dangers exist in the use of public access facilities. Risks can be grouped into dangers from staff, from strangers, and from the open "window" that certain Web sites and e-mail systems inadvertently create. Most of these dangers can be eliminated or greatly reduced through carefully prepared and enforced policies about passwords and computer use. Others can be controlled through software and hardware devices. System security is one of the most difficult—and perhaps the most important part of the Information Technology (IT) manager's job. But security cannot be only the IT manager's job. It is important that the Principal Investigator ensures that the entire research team understands that system security is everybody's job. The Internet can be a tremendously valuable source of information. It can also be the vehicle through which research databases are compromised, damaged, or destroyed. System security requires a whole other system, including software, hardware, policies, and an educated and aware research team. In this chapter, the sources of danger to the research team and its data are identified and methods for protecting against each danger are presented.

SOURCES OF DANGER

Viruses and Worms

The Internet is a window to the outside world. Researchers may use that window to access a wealth of information and to communicate among various sites where members of the research team collect data and do the work of the research project. Unfortunately, that window can also predispose the team's system and databases to viruses and worms. Almost everyone has heard about the damage that computer "viruses" can do to vital information in computer databases. A specialized form of virus called a "worm" can also enter through certain Web sites and e-mail windows and cause considerable damage.

The computer virus. A computer virus is a piece of programming code secretly attached to some innocuous item of mail or certain pages, games, or other types of programs downloaded from the Internet. There are a variety of ways that virus programmers have found to attach viruses to seemingly innocent items on the Internet. By far, e-mail has produced the most prolific spread of computer viruses. A few viruses (like the old "Happy Birthday" virus) have been designed to just send silly messages. Most, however, are designed to do two things. First, they typically are designed to spread rapidly through as many computer systems as possible—usually by attaching to the recipient's e-mail system and automatically sending themselves to every other person listed in the recipient's e-mail address book. Second, they typically damage the recipients programs, data files, or system files. Some cause so much damage that the only way to recover is to reformat the hard drive, thus losing all programs, data, and information on the hard drive.

Recently, members of various public and private discussion groups (that use listserv technology) have complained that some malicious virus programmers have joined the private groups specifically to spread their virus programs through the discussion groups. For those who consider creating a private discussion group to promote communication within the research team, having rules about virus protection, and strictly restricting group membership may offer some protection against viruses spread through discussion groups.

Computer worms. The word, "worm" can have two meanings in cyberspeech. The good meaning of a "worm" is a form of permanent, high-density storage called *Write Once, Read Many* disk. The bad meaning of worm is a specialized form of computer virus that tends not to do immediate damage to the hard drive. Rather, it continually replicates itself on the hard drive. In so doing, it takes up increasing amounts of space on the hard drive until the entire hard drive is filled up. At first, it typically overwrites parts of data and program files. In some cases, it is designed to immediately start overwriting files so that the files become riddled with "holes," almost as if a worm has eaten its way through the user's programs and data files. Worms can be very hard to discover because they often cause damage so subtly that it is weeks or even months before the user realizes that the system has a serious problem. It can take the information services (IS) people quite a while to correctly diagnose the problem and then clean the system—not to mention finding all other infected systems to which the worm has been sent, and cleaning up that damage too. Early effects of a worm invasion may include the system speed becoming noticeably compromised, programs that run, but certain features do not work, or formerly good data files suddenly having damaged parts. Ultimately, if not stopped, the worm can damage everything on the hard drive.

Damage From Viruses and Worms. Viruses and worms most typically get into a computer system through e-mail. Unfortunately, some of the most useful features of e-mail are the very facilities that make e-mail such a popular target of virus and worm programmers. The ability to have an address book to keep frequent contact information creates a vulnerability for e-mail systems. The ability to attach programs and documents to e-mail is one of the most important facilities for users. Researchers may need to send each other questions about aspects of the research, such as subject inclusion/exclusion procedures, research reports, data files, reports of adverse reactions to an experimental treatment, updates to a research protocol, reliability findings, or any other information that needs to be communicated to the research team. It can also save considerable expense in copying and typing costs to be able to send documents via e-mail.

Loss of the ability to send e-mail attachments would certainly reduce the value of e-mail tremendously. However, e-mail attachments are not easily scanned by the server's anti-virus software and thus are an attractive target for malicious virus programmers. Due to the danger of viruses, many university systems now ban all e-mail with attachments that are executable programs. The following file extensions on attachments are cause for great concern (and many are banned by university mail server systems): .EXE, .COM, .SYS, .OVL, .PRG, and .MNU. A virus is a program, and thus it needs an executable file name.

Sadly, many people need to send executable programs to each other, and the virus programmers have destroyed that option for thousands of innocent users. Researchers may need to go outside the university system if they need to send executable files. Executable files may include programs to install on a laptop so that data collectors in the field directly enter subject responses into the computer rather than on a paper data collection instrument. Depending upon the programming, the data collector may need to send an executable file to send the data back to the research office. In these cases, the research team may need to use commercial e-mail systems to send executable files to each other.

In addition to e-mail, viruses can get into systems through diskettes or CDs that have old, infected files on them. Diskettes or CDs may be infected if they contain game programs purchased through Internet advertisers. Worse, infection is common if programs were directly downloaded freeware through Internet discussion boards, chat rooms, or Internet bulletin boards. The best advice is *never* download an executable program from the Internet. Or if a program file must be downloaded, download it onto a diskette, zip drive, or other storage medium that can be isolated from the research computers. A virus detection program can then be executed on the disk, CD, or zip drive prior to opening the program. Some facilities keep a PC that is not connected in any way to the rest of the system for the purpose of downloading and using potentially infected programs. That way, if the program is infected, it may cause damage to the isolated computer, but not to the entire network. This is extremely similar to quarantining a person infected with a highly contagious disease. In both cases, an effective quarantine keeps the infection from spreading beyond the individual person or computer.

At the time of this printing, it is fairly safe to download and print documents and non-executable pages from university, governmental, and legitimate corporate Internet sites (so long as copyright laws are respected). However, downloading games and other types of executable programs is extremely risky. The risk is lessened if the researcher knows who created the executable programs. Since most people enjoy computer games; it is not unusual for staff to download games during slow work times. Unfortunately, many computer systems have become infected with computer viruses from this kind of activity. The most serious concern with having Internet access through the research project computers is that a virus could enter the research computers through the Internet and damage or compromise the programs and data files.

A virus can damage not only the recipient's computer, but also any other computer linked to the computer that first received the virus. As a result, a whole university information system could be irreparably damaged from a virus that entered via an e-mail message to a desktop computer in the research office. If the timing is particularly bad—for example, the virus enters just before a major system backup procedure—the virus might end up incorporated into the backup storage medium. In this instance, the server hard drive might have to be erased and reloaded to rid the system of the virus. Otherwise, backup drives might continue to reinfect the computer until the system administrator discovers all instances of the virus and destroys them. In the past few years, it has not been uncommon for major computer facilities to have to take the whole system down once or twice a year to clean out a virus that has infected hundreds of the PCs in the system. Unfortunately, it is not unusual for one or two office computers to be missed in the general cleanup. When these users start their system, the entire computer system may get reinfected. Another day or two can be lost as the IS employees try to remove the virus a second time.

Trojan Horses

In the old Greek epic tales, the city-state of Troy (in present day Turkey) was at war with the city-state of Sparta (in Greece). Troy had excellent city gates and even after 10 years of siege, the Spartans could not breach the walls. The Spartans, pretending to surrender, built an enormous wooden horse as a "cease-fire" gift to the City of Troy and left it, apparently unguarded, outside Troy's city gates. The people of Troy brought the horse into their city. Unbeknownst to the Trojan people, inside the horse were Spartan soldiers. At night after the Trojans were asleep, the soldiers quietly got out of the horse and opened the gates of Troy and the city was then destroyed by the Spartan army.

In the context of computer systems, a Trojan horse is defined as "any malicious, security-breaking program that is disguised as something benign" (Lo, 2003). Thus, a researcher may accidentally download a "Trojan horse" while downloading what appears to be an innocent, highly desirable program but which hides a serious threat. While a Trojan horse may merely hide a virus or worm, the most serious threat is that it will open a remote access port into the researcher's computer.

A secret remote access port (often called a backdoor) is created when a malicious outsider (cracker) sends programming with an apparently benign program that allows the outsider access into the researcher's computer. It is possible that the outsider merely wants to use the processing power of the researcher's computer to perform work. More likely, however, the cracker will steal passwords and credit card numbers, or maliciously damage the programs and data on the hard drive.

Computer Spam

The general meaning of spam in the world of e-mail is any unsolicited and unwanted e-mail. More specifically, when an unwanted item of e-mail is sent repeatedly so that the user's mailbox is literally filled up with these repetitive and unwanted messages, the recipient is said to have been spammed. Spam is defined as flooding a newsgroup, discussion group, or e-mail users with many copies of the same article, item, or e-mail. (Muller, 2003; Southwick & Falk, 1998). Some programs have been written to repeatedly replicate an e-mail message and send it in an infinite loop[1] to all members of a facility's address book. The term "spam" has also been used to mean any unsolicited e-mail, and especially advertisement e-mail. Spam can quickly fill up a user's e-mail box so that no legitimate e-mail can be received or sent.

Spam may also contain a virus. What this means is that when the victim opens the spam e-mail message, it attaches to the recipient's address book and sends itself to every person listed. Unfortunately, it doesn't send just one copy. It continues to send the same message repeatedly—in an infinite loop (an infinite loop means that the program orders a command to be carried out, but at the end, it does not tell the computer to stop and go back to the user for a new command. Instead, it orders the computer to go back to the beginning of the command sequence and start executing the same command again. When the command is to send an e-mail message to everybody in the address book, it does not take long for thousands of e-mail messages to be generated). (An infinite loop means the program orders a command to be carried out, but at the end, it does not tell the computer to stop and go back to the user for a new command. Instead, it orders the computer to go back to the beginning of the command sequence and start executing the same command again. When the command is to send an e-mail message to everybody in the address book, it does not take long for thousands of e-mail messages to be generated). Such a program has no end point. It keeps resending the same e-mail to everybody until the e-mail system becomes overwhelmed and crashes (Levine, 2003). It may also end if the amount of allocated storage space for e-mail is exceeded. (Both outgoing and incoming e-mails have to be stored on the server until deleted). When the user's e-mail box is filled with spam, the user can receive no legitimate e-mail. It often takes hours to delete all the spam out of both the inbox and outbox. As of this writing, there are no U.S. Federal laws against spam (Sorkin, 2003). Several laws have been proposed for the 2003–2004 legislative year, but as of this printing, none have been enacted.

Hackers and Crackers

The word "hackers" originally meant someone who was very interested in personal computers and explored the capabilities of these machines. However, over time, the word has come to have a more sinister meaning. Today, most people think of a hacker as a person who directly breaks into other people's computers for the purpose of stealing private information or causing damage to files and programs. Strictly, such a person should be called a *cracker* because he or she "cracks" into another's computer. A cracker gains entry into private computers by using the Internet as a pathway. The portal of entry is usually a known weakness in the e-mail or operating system. Unfortunately, many people fail to protect their passwords and some crackers get into systems through a Trojan horse and steal the person's passwords.

Human nature being what it is, people often are extraordinarily careless with passwords. Passwords are hard for many people to remember. In many installations, the IS personnel require that users change their password every 3 months or so, which can contribute to increased difficulty remembering a password. Assignment of nonsense passwords composed of a random mixture of letters and numbers can further contribute to this problem. When a password is forgotten, it can be time consuming to obtain a new one from the IS department.

To be sure the passwords are available to the legitimate users, users often write them down somewhere. That somewhere is often on or near the computer where they are convenient for any casual passerby to inspect—and later use to hack into a hospital or university's computer. Other passwords have been compromised when a user taped it to his/her own computer at home. Friends of teenaged children have used passwords to hack into a work computer "for fun." The only real solution is to design a people-friendly security system. How to do that will be addressed in the section on how to overcome the dangers.

Inadvertent Security Lapses

Offering Internet access in a research office is typically provided on the same PC that the staff uses to access research databases. Staff may inadvertently infect the system with viruses through unwise downloading activities, through opening e-mail with infected attachments, and by bringing in infected diskettes from home and using them on the research office computers without first running them through an anti-virus program. Staff may leave their passwords in places that hackers can find them. Staff may give each other their passwords for convenience. The purpose is never to violate security. But security is often extremely inconvenient to computer users. They may feel that the computers should have been designed and implemented to promote their efforts to get their work done. But security policies and practices sometimes impede efforts to work efficiently. When computer security interferes with work, people may bypass security protocols.

METHODS TO PROTECT AGAINST THE DANGERS OF THE INTERNET

There are five types of security that may be used in the research office: isolation, anti-virus protection programs, hardware devices, password protections, and security policies. Confidential databases must be protected against accidental damage or loss of the data, unauthorized access to confidential files, corruption of the files by viruses and worms, and damage to the files by crackers. Different risks require different security approaches, and some security approaches will protect against a variety of hazards.

Isolation

The safest research data files are in a computer that has absolutely no Internet or intranet access. If it is at all possible, one computer should be set aside as the research data repository and data analysis machine. This computer is therefore isolated. It will contain the raw data files, a data analysis program such as SPSS or SAS, the analysis files (research data stored in a format readable by the data analysis program), and an office package that includes a word processor, graphics package, and perhaps a database management system and spreadsheet. This computer is not linked to the Internet or to the institution's computer network. There is no phone modem, Ethernet link, or in fact, any other link between this computer and any other system. Its only input devices are the keyboard and mouse, a CD-ROM, and perhaps a diskette or USB drive. Viruses, worms, and Trojan horses cannot get in except through the portable storage devices (disks, CDs, or USB drives). If the storage devices are new and used only for saving back-ups of the research data there is no danger. If they are used to bring in new research data from distant data collection sites, they should be run through a virus scanner program prior to use in the isolated computer.

Anti-virus protection programs. Sometimes it is not feasible or even desirable to have the research data on an isolated computer. So every computer needs anti-virus software. Several companies have developed and marketed software designed to detect viruses, worms and Trojan horses, and to block them before they can infect the system. The two most popular products in this line include the Norton and MacAffee anti-virus programs (both are copyrighted). Both products have Web sites designed to let product purchasers update their products and provide lots of helpful information about how to keep one's system clean and free of viruses. Other freeware such as Ad-Alert by Lavasoft company (http://www.lavasoftusa.com/) or Spybot by PepiMK Software Company (http://security.kolla.de/) are designed to detect and remove secret files left on the computer during Internet sessions. Every computer should have anti-virus program protection. Even if the computer is an isolated computer, programs and the research data itself must be entered in some way and this often means diskettes or CDs used in another computer and brought to the isolated research computer. Those media need to be checked by an anti-virus program before any data or files are downloaded.

Hardware Security Solutions

Biometric devices can be used to protect access to the computer programs and files. A biometric device is equipment that can read physical characteristics that are unique to an individual. Some read a fingerprint or palm print. Some read voice prints and others do a scan of the retina of the eye or the entire face (O'Shea & Lee, 1999a). Formerly, these devices were extremely expensive and limited to use in high security environments, such as defense department, CIA, and NASA computers. Today, they can be acquired for under $50 per computer (O'Shea

& Lee, 1999b). O'Shea and Lee mentioned that many users are resistant to these devices from fear of new technology or from distaste for finger and palm printing as more a criminal detection technology than a computer security technology. However, these devices are much more convenient than having to remember frequently changed, nonsense passwords. Relief from the inconvenience of password protocols makes these devices highly desirable in a research office that contains confidential, personally identifiable subject information.

Policy Protections

The most basic protection any Research Office must have is to write policies pertaining to staff behavior. The policies must be taught in orientation, reviewed annually or semi-annually, and enforced vigorously. In some hospitals, the penalty for compromising one's password is a suspension for the first violation and termination for the second. Research offices would do well to have similar policies due to the extremely confidential nature of patient information contained in many research databases.

The Principal Investigator (PI) is ultimately responsible for the security of the research database. Thus, it is primarily the PI who must be sure that computer security policies are enforced. There should be regular reminders to the staff of the danger to the entire system—and, of course, to subject confidentiality—of any lapses in staff behavior with respect to computer security. Policy should address keeping the room locked, password security, and bringing in unauthorized storage devices that could contaminate the research computer(s) with a virus or worm.

Even if the computer is not linked in any way to a network or to the Internet, access to the computer itself should be restricted. Keeping the computer in a locked office is the first level of security. Policies should state that staff should not leave the office unlocked unless someone is physically in that office whenever it is unlocked. Thus, when a member of the research staff leaves the office for a break, lunch, or a meeting, a policy should be in place that requires the staff to lock the office, regardless of the expected duration of the absence.

If biometric devices are not used, passwords are the next type of security that can be used to protect against unauthorized access to research databases. Policies should address the need to protect the secrecy of passwords.

Password security policies. If access to the computer itself and its files is not protected with a biometric device, then passwords should be required first to access the computer itself, and then separate passwords should be used to protect access to confidential research data files. This means there should be a two-level password (typically called a userID and password) required to load even the operating system when the computer is first turned on. Then the system should be programmed to require a separate password to gain access to the research data files. In fact, it is possible to give users different levels of access, depending upon what files and even variables their job requires them to use. Policy should require that passwords be changed on a regular basis, and whenever an employee leaves the research team, that person's passwords should be immediately cancelled.

The most important policy pertaining to computer system security is the policy demanding that people keep their personal passwords secret. Posting passwords in the computer office next to the computer renders all password protection strategies ineffective. When people reveal their passwords to others—even to coworkers, nobody can be really sure who signed on using that password. It may give access to personally identifiable subject data to someone who is not authorized to see that information. Thus, it makes protecting the confidentiality of private health data impossible. Therefore, strict policies about keeping one's password secret are an important part of the system security plan.

Firewall. Having the research computer isolated from all outside links is not feasible when the research data must be collected from distant sites and sent via the Internet to the main research database. The benefits to distributed research sites of having the research computer networked through the Internet are so great that a different software protection approach has typically been adopted. Often, the central research database is located within a university or hospital that has installed a firewall to protect the entire system from problems. A firewall may be a hardware device that contains protective software, or it may be strictly a software approach (Webopedia, 2003). In either case, it is designed to block access to the information system by unauthorized persons and to identify and block hidden code (which is almost always a virus) in messages or downloads from the Internet. A firewall sits at the junction between the internal network and the link from the outside computer world into the private network.

The software in a firewall examines all traffic entering or leaving the private network to see if it meets criteria specified by the IS programmers. If an outside hacker does not have a legitimate UserID and password (or a recognized physical pattern from a physical recognition system), entry is blocked by the firewall. Another way firewalls often filter out unauthorized persons is to check the ID of the computer the hacker is using. As part of setting up a password or physical recognition system, the system administrators can also program the system to limit access from only identified computers. When authorized users want to enter from home, part of the setup procedure involves them registering their computer's unique identifier with the firewall software. Even with a legitimate UserID and Password, the hacker will be unsuccessful unless he or she is using the legitimate user's computer.

There can be some real disadvantages to firewalls. Some were designed to allow the user to passively view all Internet sites that contain information, but blocks all interactive sites. If distant research data collection sites need to be able to interact with the central research computer, the firewall may block such communication. Some firewalls allow users to print Internet pages, but not to download anything. This can be a real problem if it forces people to retype pages of information. For those interested in learning more about firewalls, there is an excellent introductory article (Vicomsoft, 2003) about firewalls at the following URL:http://www.vicomsoft.com/knowledge/reference/firewalls1. html?track=internal.

Firewalls cannot protect against misbehavior or deliberate sabotage by someone who has stolen the passwords of a legitimate user. This is another reason why policies against revealing passwords are so important—and why use of biometrics is better than using passwords. Additionally, sabotage by terminated employees has been a serious problem for some companies. Almost anybody can have high tech skills today. The PI should not assume that an employee does not have well developed programming and Internet capabilities just because the employee is not an IT professional. Indeed, some of the most successful hackers in history have been high school children.

The simple activity of terminating passwords, biometric identifiers, and changing UserID codes for a department whenever an employee terminates (either voluntarily or involuntarily) is the most basic safety procedure for any competent IS department. In fact, if an employee is to be terminated involuntarily, it is usually a good procedure for the PI to have that employee's access terminated during or immediately before the termination interview. It is much safer to give terminated employees 2 weeks termination pay free than to give them 2 weeks notice and risk compromise of the computer system during that time. This seems cruel because very few terminated employees will actually commit acts of sabotage. However, one disgruntled employee with some sophisticated computer skills can do enormous damage to a research database.

CONCLUSION

There are potential dangers to Internet access in any area. Internet access carries with it the risk of opening the door to viruses and worms, the danger that e-mail accounts will be flooded with spam, and that staff will inadvertently let hackers in through carelessness with passwords. In addition, employees can personally compromise their jobs through unwise use of e-mail and by visiting inappropriate Internet sites while at work.

Although no protection scheme is perfect, a variety of hardware and software tools have been developed to help companies protect the confidentiality and security of information systems. Policies properly written and strictly enforced can reduce incidences of employees becoming careless with passwords. Physical recognition devices can make passwords obsolete and offer a much higher degree of security for the company's information system. One approach that has been used to both provide Internet access and yet keep the information system isolated from the dangers of the Internet is to have Internet access provided only through special, isolated computers that have no connection to the computers containing research data. That solution has not been adopted often, because most IS managers are now implementing firewall technology to control access to their internal computer network. Firewalls create constraints and barriers that may limit the benefits of Internet use.

REFERENCES

Levine, J. *Why is spam bad? Coalition Against Unsolicited Commercial E-Mail (CAUCE).* Retrieved August 31, 2003 from http://spam.abuse.net/ overview/spambad.shtml

Lo, J. (2003). *Trojan horse attacks. Internet Relay Chat (IRC) Security Pages.* Available at: http://www.irchelp.org/irchelp/security/trojan.html

Muller, S. H. What is Spam? Coalition Against Unsolicited Commercial E-Mail (CAUCE). Retrieved August 31, 2003, from http://spam.abuse.net/overview/whatisspam.shtml

O'Shea, T., & Lee, M. (1999a). Biometric authentication management. *Network Computing.* Available at: http://www.networkcomputing.com/ 1026/1026f2.html

O'Shea, T., & Lee, M. (1999b). BioNetrix Suite covers all the bases—Product review. *Network Computing.* Available at: http://www.networkcomputing.com/ 1026/1026f22.html?ls=NCJS_1026bt

Sorkin, D. (2003). Summary of bills introduced in 108th Congress. *Spam Laws: United States: Federal Laws: 108th Congress.* http://www.spamlaws.com/federal/list108.html

Southwick, S., & Falk, J. D. (1998). *The Net Abuse FAQ. Coalition Against Unsolicited Commercial E-Mail (CAUCE).* Available at: http://www.cybernothing.org/ faqs/net-abuse-faq.html#2.1

Vicomsoft, Ltd. (2003). *Firewall Q and A. Vicomsoft Ltd. Knowledge Share White Papers.* Available at: http:// www.vicomsoft.com/knowledge/reference/ firewalls1.html?track=internal

Webopedia. (2003). *Firewall.* Webopedia: Online Encyclopedia Dedicated to Computer Technology. Jupiter Media Corporation. Available at: http:// www.webopedia.com/TERM/f/firewall.html

Part **III**

Teaching Research Online

Chapter 15

Using the Internet in Undergraduate Research Education

Carol Holdcraft

U ndergraduate education in nursing research provides the practicing nurse with the basic knowledge and skills necessary to read and comprehend published research studies for application to practice (American Association of Colleges of Nursing [AACN], 1998). As a practice profession, nursing is moving away from tradition and authority as the basis for practice toward evidence-based practice. Thus, nurses must learn the language and processes of research, read and understand research that is pertinent to their practice areas, and determine if the research is credible and of significance to practice. Teaching nursing research to undergraduate students is both a necessity and a challenge. Undergraduate nursing students are often more focused on learning the specific knowledge and skills needed for clinical practice. Courses in nursing research are sometimes perceived as dry and uninteresting (Ax & Kincade, 2001) by the young student who is eager to take care of patients to become a "real nurse." Undergraduate nursing students need to actively participate in learning about research; they respond best to a variety of teaching methods (Dobratz, 2003).

Critical thinking is one of the core competencies relevant to nursing research education (AACN). Baccalaureate prepared nurses are expected to "apply research-based knowledge from nursing and the sciences as the basis for practice" (p. 10). To fully implement a professional role, the nurse is expected to base practice on current research as well as to participate in research (AACN, 1998). In a study of trends in registered nurse education prepared for the National League for Nursing, Adams, Murdock, Valiga, McGinnis & Worfertz (n.d.) found that informatics and computers, as well as evidence-based practice, were two of six topics that were getting more emphasis in 1999 as compared to 1994. These two topics were also expected to have even more emphasis in 2004.

The Internet provides ways to enhance traditional nursing research classroom courses. There are many resources available that can be used to bring the research topics to life and make them more vibrant and interesting for undergraduate students. In addition, nursing research is a course that is well suited to being wholly delivered via the Internet since it typically does not include clinical experiences. This chapter identifies the research skills that are important for undergraduate education in nursing research and how those skills can be fostered using the Internet. Internet resources are described including evidence-based standards. Teaching strategies for using the Internet to enhance the knowledge, skills, and attitudes of undergraduate nursing students are described.

EVIDENCE-BASED PRACTICE

The gap between research evidence and nursing practice has long been the source of consternation among nurse researchers and other nursing leaders. Research utilization by nurses was a subject for research (Brett, 1987; Coyle & Sokop, 1990) and several programs to enhance the movement of tested innovations into the practice arena have been implemented (Krueger, Nelson, & Wolanin, 1978; Horsley, Crane, & Bingle, 1978; Bostrom & Wise, 1994; Rutledge & Donaldson, 1995). More recently, the term evidenced-based practice has gained prominence as a necessary requirement for quality improvement to occur in the fast-paced health care arena. Evidence-based nursing requires the skills to be able to define the nursing care problem, skills to search for, access, and evaluate research literature, and determine its applicability to the practice problem (Kessenich, Guyatt, & DiCenso, 1997). Evidence-based nursing is a broader philosophy of learning meant to guide nurses in clinical decision-making throughout their professional careers (Kessenich, et al.). In addition to teaching nursing students the skills required for evidence-based practice, the expectation must be carried throughout clinical nursing courses with enthusiastic clinical faculty who are adept at role modeling the value of evidence-based practice. The Agency for Healthcare Research and Quality (AHRQ, 2003) convenes expert panels to summarize the state of the art on clinical topics of interest and then develop clinical practice guidelines. The National Guideline Clearinghouse (NGC) is one resource for evidence-based guidelines. The NGC's mission is to provide a means for obtaining objective, detailed information on clinical practice guidelines so that up-to-date guidelines will be used in practice (NGC, 2003). Internet resources, such as those available through NGC, provide useful information, quickly and reliably, to update practice.

UNDERGRADUATE NURSING RESEARCH SKILLS

Graduates of baccalaureate nursing programs are not expected to take on the role of designing and carrying out independent research projects. They are expected to be "consumers" of nursing research, able to read and comprehend research for the purpose of extending their knowledge base and making decisions about changes to their practice. Baccalaureate graduates are expected to value research for its contributions to the advancement of the discipline of nursing, so that they will support the efforts of nurse researchers through subject recruitment, protocol implementation, or data collection in clinical research projects. Nurses are expected, no matter what their level of education, to know about and be able to explain to their clients, friends, and families about the latest research on health and health care treatments. Especially when the media highlights on a new article on health research, nurses are expected to explain to the public what they should do for their personal health based on this new knowledge. Without a grounding in basic research terminology, methods, and skills, nurses would be as bewildered as the public with the new information. The research skills of literature searching, reading and comprehension, critiquing for credibility, and determining the applicability for practice are all ones that should be part of baccalaureate nursing education.

Literature Searching

A key skill that is required to be a successful baccalaureate student is to be able to successfully search the literature for relevant articles to answer questions about clinical practice. French (1998) suggested that participating in a process of locating, appraising, and synthesizing research evidence may be as useful a skill as the former practice of having students participate in a faculty member's research. The process involves defining the clinical question that needs an evidence-based answer (much like defining a problem for a research proposal). The student learns to identify the appropriate terms to guide the search by defining the problem, identifying possible variables, and consulting the key term thesaurus of the database. Collaboration with a health-science librarian for teaching basic literature search skills to undergraduate students has been effective (Shorten, Wallace & Crookes, 2001). The earlier in the nursing curriculum that literature searching skills are taught, the more students can use the skill to find appropriate information throughout their program. More advanced searching skills can be introduced as part of the undergraduate nursing research course for the purpose of conducting an integrative review to answer a specific clinical question. In an online program for RN-BSN completion students, faculty incorporated a group assignment to develop a research proposal for two community agencies as part of the community health clinical experience (Cannon & Boswell, 2001). Students were able to develop skills needed by the professional nurse and use the basic literature searching skills developed in prior nursing research courses to meet a need requested by the community agencies.

A web-based tutorial on search procedures is a good starting point for learning the basics of literature searching. (See for instance the PubMed Tutorial from the National Library of Medicine Web site.) Most students find that working one-to-one with an experienced reference librarian on a specific question allows the students to refine and improve their literature searching techniques. Many libraries have added innovative ways to access the help of a research librarian, such as online tutorials, frequently asked questions, e-mail a reference question, librarian chats, as well as the traditional phone or walk-in access to the reference librarians.

Reading and Comprehending Research

For many undergraduate students, reading research studies is among the most difficult reading they have encountered in college. Not only do they have to negotiate what seems like a foreign language, but they also are faced with reading that requires a knowledge of statistics. As Bean (1996) so aptly puts it,

"Armed with a yellow highlighter but with no apparent strategy for using it and hampered by lack of knowledge of how skilled readers actually go about reading, our students are trying to catch marlin with the tools of a worm fisherman" (p. 133).

One strategy for helping students learn to read research is to describe for them how you approach a new research article (Bean). Most accomplished researchers start with the title and note the variables that are identified there. Next they will read the abstract to see the research purpose, question, and theoretical framework. A quick skim of the introduction gives the experienced research reader a sense of how the author has framed the research problem. At this point, many researchers will skip back to the findings, followed by the discussion and conclusions. Only when it appears that this is a study of interest will the experienced research reader go back to the methodology section to carefully review how the study was conducted and make judgments about its merit.

Another helpful strategy to teach undergraduate students how to read research is to share your method of marking the text and taking notes (Bean, 1996). A scanned article with the teacher's marginal notations and underlining can be posted in Adobe Acrobat Reader for the students to see and with an assignment to read and mark their own research article. Ask students to "translate" a difficult passage within a research article into their own words as another strategy to determine if the student comprehends the text.

Critiquing Research

In order to be a discerning consumer of research, the practicing nurse must be able to comprehend the strengths and weaknesses of published research. The skill of critiquing research is a higher level analytical skill that requires comprehension, comparison to standards or criteria, and the ability to weigh the overall merits of a study. While the basics of this skill are appropriate to baccalaureate nursing students, continuing development of the skill should occur in graduate and even postgraduate education and experience. A written critique of a single research report is a common assignment in baccalaureate nursing research education. It is favored by faculty because it requires the student to demonstrate their understanding of the research report as well as their comprehension of numerous principles of good research practice. Many undergraduate research textbooks are organized with guidelines or criteria for critiquing included in each chapter of the text, with a culminating chapter that discusses the overall process of research critique (Polit, Beck, & Hungler, 2001; LoBiondo-Wood, & Haber, 2002; Nieswiadomy, 2001). Although the formal research critique is a useful outcome product for an undergraduate research course, a less time-subsuming process such as a check sheet may be used later in the nursing curriculum to foster the critiquing skills.

An innovative alternative to the usual format of research critiques was developed to address the problems of students focusing on parts, but not the whole of a research study, and the tendency of students to be overly critical of research. Shellenbarger (1998) had students write their critique in the form of a letter to the researcher. This assignment forced students to critically evaluate the overall strengths and weaknesses to produce a balanced professional letter. The "Dear Researcher" assignment was less time intensive for faculty to grade as well as a useful learning strategy for students (Shellenbarger).

STRATEGIES FOR TEACHING RESEARCH

Many creative strategies for teaching nursing research have been reported in the literature over the years; however limited evaluation studies have been done with adequate controls for validity (Porter, 2001). Nevertheless, some examples of narrative reports of teaching strategies can be shared for the purpose of encouraging faculty to continue the quest for ways to make this important nursing education area more interesting for students. The situated learning model (McLellan, 1996) served as a basis for developing a continuing education workshop titled "Gourmet Research" for practicing nurses (Gieselman, Stark, & Farruggia, 2000). The gourmet cooking theme provided humor and interest to an otherwise dry topic. Wisneski (1998) noted from personal experience that minority students were more skeptical of the value of nursing research and less trusting of research findings than students from majority cultures. She suggested that teaching strategies such as case methods and journal responses are useful to help minority students express their concerns so they can learn basic research concepts and can come to appreciate the importance of nursing research to professional practice.

The Internet is becoming a popular method for delivering nursing courses, particularly to RN-BSN completion students and graduate students. For undergraduate nursing prelicensure students, the requirements for psychomotor skills and clinical experiences has meant that Internet courses are more often used only for nonclinical courses. Nursing research is typically taught as a nonclinical course in most baccalaureate nursing programs so it can be taught via the Internet even to prelicensure students. Woo and Kimmick (2000) found no differences in outcomes for graduate nursing students who took an Internet version compared to those who took the usual lecture version of a nursing research course. Their students were equally satisfied in both versions of the course. The Internet students did report higher stimulation of learning than the classroom students. However, Woo and Kimmick noted that a limitation of their study was the high percentage of Internet students (73%) who reported attending at least a third of the classroom lectures.

The hyperlearning process model (Jeffries, 2000) was used to design a Web-based nursing research course (Sternberger, 2002a). Students learned general principles of nursing research through assigned text readings, slide show presentations, research articles, and Internet Web sites in each of ten course modules. Process activities were used to allow students to interact with the materials and get feedback on their comprehension. Each module of the research course had a written assignment or quiz to test students' critical thinking about key concepts. Students demonstrated their ability to synthesize and apply research concepts through an assigned critique of a published research article. Discussion forums were used to help students apply research concepts to professional practice. An example given was the use of Internet links to the Nuremberg Code, the Belmont Report, the Tuskegee syphilis study, and other sites, to prepare for discussion on a research ethics forum where they related a site of interest to a research article that had ethical considerations not fully discussed by the study's authors (Sternberger, 2002a). In this way, students related the information to their experience as nurses. As part of her development of activities to help the nursing research content "come alive" for students, Sternberger (2002b) revised a strategy that had originally been described by Thiel (1987) and amplified by Morrison-Beedy and Cote-Arsenault (2000) as "The Cookie Experiment" and developed "The Great Music Experiment" to be feasible in an online format. The Great Music Experiment is available through the Merlot Project, http://www.merlot.org/Home.po, which is a sharing resource for educators. A search of available topics in the Merlot project turned up a Research Answers and Questions game, and several statistical topics that can be used by faculty teaching online research courses.

Nursing faculty have shared creative ways to integrate nursing research into clinical courses in the curriculum of undergraduate programs as a way to increase students' understanding of research concepts as well as to appreciate the clinical relevance of nursing research. Moss and Nesbitt (2003) collaborated to integrate research concepts across two courses in a master's curriculum, but their ideas are also relevant to undergraduate education. In a community health course, students were given the assignment to interview two clients with chronic health problems about their perceived health status and quality of life. The students learned about the qualitative method, interviewing and transcribing techniques, and obtaining participant consent. Reflections and discussion of insights gained about quality of life and health was done during the community health course. Students in the nursing research course then analyzed data, and the project became the example for many research concepts discussed throughout the course (Moss & Nesbitt, 2003).

A research course and adult health clinical nursing course were linked in another study using collaborative learning projects (Kenty, 2001). Each group collaboratively identified a practice problem on the clinical units. Students worked independently to search the nursing literature to develop a reference list of practice innovation research reports. Faculty assisted the students to select a nursing innovation with an outcome measure that would be feasible in the clinical setting. Students then used a case study method to implement the practice innovation and evaluate its effectiveness. Group presentations at the end of the term were used to present the practice problem, critique of selected research reports, and presentation of the implementation and evaluation of practice innovations. Faculty reported that these activities served as good discussion points for various research concepts and helped students synthesize knowledge and understand the importance of evidence-based practice.

Nursing faculty introduced a research utilization component to a senior level maternity/pediatrics clinical course (Radjenovic & Chally, 1998). Faculty selected research topics where there was a sufficient research base and staff nurses in the clinical setting identified the topic as a practice problem area. Each student used a structured research critique form to review and critique two research articles. Faculty led a seminar to organize and summarize findings into an integrative review. Comparative discussions about current practice, feasibility, risk assessment, and organizational readiness for change helped students understand the whole research utilization process. Students prepared a poster presentation that summarized their comparative evaluation process and made recommendations for practice and research. Posters could be shared with nursing staff as well as at research symposia.

Senior BSN students who had completed a previous nursing research course participated in a community health research project (Neafsey & Shellman, 2002). Students were trained in the research protocol and then delivered the interactive computer education program about drug interactions to elderly home-care clients. Students participated in subject recruitment, delivery of the intervention, and collection of data from participants. The senior nursing students with clients participating in the research project gained more knowledge about drug interactions in the elderly and reported an increase in confidence and skills in the research process (Neafsey & Shellman, 2002). In another strategy to involve students in a research project, the nursing students' attitudes toward nursing research were improved by adding an opportunity to participate in collecting oral history interviews of nurses (Druggleby, 1998).

RESOURCES

There are many useful resources available on the Internet to help faculty teach undergraduate nursing students about nursing research in a way that inspires and educates. For instance, the home page for the National Institute for Nursing Research (2003) can be used to show students the history of NINR and how it came into being, as well as to direct their attention to the latest priorities for nursing research funding. Students who explore this site can learn about the connections with government legislation, members of the National Advisory Council for Nursing Research, and diversity and resources for minority students and researchers. Press releases on the NINR home page show students how nursing research findings can be announced to the media in ways that share important new information with the public. A link off of the resource button can take students to the PubMed Web site (National Library of Medicine, 2002) where they can go through the PubMed Tutorial.

To help students see that nurses in other countries are interested in nursing research, introduce them to the Royal Windsor Society of Nurse Researchers (2003). This site has many useful online tutorials as well as a nursing research jeopardy game where students can challenge their knowledge.

REFERENCES

Adams, C. E., Murdock, J. E., Valiga, T. M., McGinnis, S., & Wolfertz, J. R. (n.d.). *Trends in registered nurse education programs: A comparison across three points in time–1994, 1999, 2004.* Prepared for the National League for Nursing. Retrieved July 1, 2003, from http://www.nln.org/aboutnln/ nurse-trends.htm

Agency for Healthcare Research and Quality. (2003, March). *Evidence-based Practice Centers.* Overview. (AHRQ Publication No. 03-P006), Agency for Healthcare Research and Quality, Rockville, MD. Retreived from http:// www.ahrq.gov/clinic/epc/

American Association of Colleges of Nursing. (1998). *The essentials of baccalaureate education for professional nursing practice.* Washington, DC: American Association of Colleges of Nursing.

Ax, S., & Kincade, E. (2001). Nursing students' perceptions of research: Usefulness, implementation and training. *Journal of Advanced Nursing, 35,* 161–170.

Bean, J. C. (1996). Engaging ideas: *The professor's guide to integrating writing, critical thinking, and active learning in the classroom.* San Francisco: Jossey-Bass.

Bostrom, J., & Wise, L. (1994). Closing the gap between research and practice. *Journal of Nursing Administration, 24,* 22–27.

Brett, J. L. L. (1987). Use of nursing practice research findings. *Nursing Research, 36,* 344–349.

Cannon, S. B., & Boswell, C. (2001). Addressing the community research needs of baccalaureate students. *Nursing and Health Care Perspectives, 22,* 194–196.

Coyle, L. A., & Sokop, A. G. (1990) Innovation adoption behavior among nurses. *Nursing Research, 39,* 176–180.

Dobratz, M. C. (2003). Putting the pieces together: Teaching undergraduate research from a theoretical perspective. *Journal of Advanced Nursing, 41,* 383–392.

Druggleby, W. (1998). Improving undergraduate nursing research education: The effectiveness of collecting and analyzing oral histories. *Journal of Nursing Education, 37,* 247–252.

French, B. (1998). Developing the skills required for evidence-based practice. *Nurse Education Today, 18,* 46–51.

Gieselman, J. A., Stark, N., & Farruggia, M. J. (2000). Implications of the situated learning model for teaching and learning nursing research. *Journal of Continuing Education in Nursing, 31,* 263–268.

Horsley, J. A., Crane, J., & Bingle, J. D. (1978). Research utilization as an organizational process. *Journal of Nursing Administration, 8,* 4–6.

Jeffries, P. R. (2000). Development and test of a model for designing interactive CD-ROMs for teaching nursing skills. *Computers in Nursing, 18,* 118–124.

Kenty, J. R. (2001). Weaving undergraduate research into practice-based experiences. *Nurse Educator, 26,* 182–186.

Kessenich, C. R., Guyatt, G. H., & DiCenso, A. (1997). Teaching nursing students evidence-based nursing. *Nurse Educator, 22,* 25–29.

Krueger, J. C., Nelson, A. H., & Wolanin, M. O. (1978). *Nursing research: Development, collaboration, and utilization.* Germantown, MD: Aspen Systems Corporation.

LoBiondo-Wood, G., & Haber, J. (2002). *Nursing research: Methods, critical appraisal, and utilization.* St. Louis: Mosby.

McLellan, H. (1996). Situated learning: Multiple perspectives. In H. McLellan (Ed.), *Situated learning perspectives* (pp. 5–17). Englewood Cliffs: Educational Technology Publications, Inc.

Morrison-Beedy, D., & Cote-Arsenault, D. (2000). The cookie experiment revisited: Broadened dimensions for teaching nursing research. *Nurse Educator, 25,* 294–296.

Moss, V., & Nesbitt, B. (2003). Research reflections. Making nursing research "real": An experiential approach. *Nurse Educator, 28,* 63–65.

National Guideline Clearinghouse. (2003). *About NCG.* Retrieved July 1, 2003, from http://www.guideline.gov/about/about.aspx

National Institute of Nursing Research. (2003). *About NINR.* Retrieved July 1, 2003, from http://www.nih.gov/ninr/

National Library of Medicine. (2002). *PubMed Tutorial.* Retrieved July 1, 2003, from http://www.nlm.nih.gov/bsd/pubmed_tutorial/ m1001.html

Neafsey, P. J., & Shellman, J. (2002). Senior nursing students' participating in a community research project: Effect on student self-efficacy and knowledge concerning drug interactions arising from self-medication in older adults. *Journal of Nursing Education, 41,* 178–181.

Nieswiadomy, R. M. (2001). *Foundations of nursing research.* Englewood Cliffs, NJ: Prentice Hall.

Polit, D. F., Beck, C. T., & Hungler, B. P. (2001). *Essentials of nursing research: Methods, appraisal, and utilization.* Philadelphia: Lippincott, Williams, & Wilkins.

Porter, E. J. (2001). Teaching undergraduate nursing research: A narrative review of evaluation studies and a typology for further research. *Journal of Nursing Education, 40,* 53–62.

Radjenovic, D., & Chally, P. S. (1998). Research utilization by undergraduate students. *Nurse Educator, 23*(2), 26–29.

Royal Windsor Society of Nurse Researchers. (2003). Retrieved July 1, 2003, from http://www.kelcom.igs.net/~nhodgins/

Rutledge, D. N., & Donaldson, N. E. (1995). Building organization capacity to engage in research utilization. *Journal of Nursing Administration, 25,* 12–16.

Shellenbarger, T. (1998). Dear researcher: An alternative to the research critique. *Journal of Nursing Education, 37,* 264–265.

Shorten, A., Wallace, M. C., & Crookes, P. A. (2001). Developing information literacy: A key to evidence-based nursing. *International Nursing Review, 48,* 86–92.

Sternberger, C. S. (2002a). Embedding a pedagogical model in the design of an online course. *Nurse Educator, 27,* 170–173.

Sternberger, C. S. (2002b). The great music experiment: Taking the cookie experiment to the Web. *Nurse Educator, 27,* 106–108.

Thiel, C. A. (1987). The cookie experiment: A creative teaching strategy. *Nurse Educator, 12,* 8–10.

Wisneski, S. M. (1998). Teaching nursing research to minority students. *ABNF Journal, 9,* 135–135.

Woo, M. A., & Kimmick, J. V. (2000). Comparison of Internet versus lecture instructional methods for teaching nursing research. *Journal of Professional Nursing, 16,* 132–139.

Chapter 16

Web-Based Graduate Research Courses

Nola Stair and Carolyn F. Waltz

Recent technological advances have created new, as well as endless, possibilities for enhancing the teaching and learning process through the use of Web-based instruction. Web-based instruction can provide new sources of content-rich learning materials as well as traditional quality education to nontraditional students.

Web-Based graduate research courses are particularly suited for online delivery, which tend to be more in-depth than undergraduate research courses. Graduate students also tend to have jobs while attending school, making online options more attractive. Due to the "anytime, anywhere" accessibility, students are able to critique research studies, conduct literature reviews, and have group discussions concerning appropriate research methodologies without being limited to set times or geographical locations. As students begin designing their own research proposals, experts from around the world can either join online discussions or appear in digitized format to share their own research findings and/or to mentor students. The availability of online datasets provides infinite opportunities to increase knowledge and skills, and extend awareness of ethical issues in health research, nursing research priorities, and new trends.

The increasing popularity of the online course delivery format accompanied by a proliferation of Web-based offerings for a variety of educational purposes including academic courses, professional development, and continuing education programs for lifelong learners has led to the establishment of policies by a number of professional organizations designed to ensure that online learning programs maintain the same standards of high quality as traditional education programs. Of particular significance are the American Association of Colleges of Nursing (AACN) *Statement on Distance Education Policies* that has been endorsed by an alliance of 14 nursing accreditation and program review bodies (AACN, 2003) and the Institute for Higher Education Policy (2000) *Quality on the Line: Benchmarks for Internet–Based Distance Education.* Existing policies and standards provide guidance for the development of Web-based research courses that are effective and sustainable and a set of criteria useful to consumers in selecting from among the many courses available to them. Common to all are standards and benchmarks in seven categories: institutional support, course development, teaching/learning, course structure, faculty support, student support, and evaluation and assessment.

INSTITUTIONAL SUPPORT

A reliable technology infrastructure and documented technology plan should be in place prior to beginning to develop and deliver Web-based distance education courses. At a minimum, the infrastructure plan should address adequate server storage and growth capacity, a courseware management system, security of user IDs and passwords, backup procedures, multimedia equipment, and identified instructional and information technology support.

In addition, an institutional committee approach is useful in determining responsible parties for coordinating registration, enrollment, and sequencing of Web-based course offerings. As enrollment in Web-based courses grows, additional planning and funding is necessary to integrate the courseware management system with the university's student information system and university electronic mail system. (Mills, Fisher, & Stair, 2001)

There are a variety of courseware management systems, ranging from no-cost solutions to expensive school-based server solutions. Key factors that will determine the selection of a courseware management system include cost, learning curve, and overall strengths/weaknesses of delivering online instruction. Table 16.1 provides a comparison of five of the most popular courseware management systems in these four areas.

Table 16.1 Comparison of Courseware Management Systems

System	Cost	Learning Curve	Strengths	Weaknesses
Blackboard	$10–25,000	Little	User-Friendly	Limited Flexibility
WebCT	$10–25,000	Significant	Abundance of Features	Complexity of Features
NiceNet	Free	Little	Hosted Off-Site	Limited Tool Set
Angel	Free	Moderate	Integrated Development Tools	Additional Per-Tool Charge
Open Source	Free	Moderate	Flexibility and Adaptability	Programming Assistance Needed

While each system typically provides tools for posting announcements, submitting assignments, adding course content, creating quizzes/exams, and communicating with students, course developers should recognize the unique capabilities that each one offers. A more in-depth comparison of online courseware management systems is available at http://www.marshall.edu/it/cit/Webct/compare/index.htm.

More than a solid technology infrastructure and courseware management system is required to develop a fully interactive and engaging Web-based course. The Southern Regional Education Board's (SREB) Distance Learning Laboratory Faculty Issues 2001 report, *Supporting Faculty in the Use of Technology: A Guide to Principles, Policies, and Implementation Strategies,* stresses the need for an instructional team and identifies the following roles as essential elements of the team's functioning:

- Instructional Designer—assists with integrating instructional technology, learning theory and strategies into the teaching/learning process and develops course materials in collaboration with the content expert and instructor.
- Graphic/Interface Designer—works with the instructional designer and instructor to create usable, functional, and visually/aesthetically appealing graphics and multimedia for course modules.

- Technical Support Personnel—provide technical support for the network, servers, hardware, software, and other resources required to seamlessly and transparently deliver Web-based instruction.
- Content Expert—provides expertise of subject matter and its proper sequencing.
- Direct Instructor—assists with developing course materials but ultimately is responsible for delivering the Web-based course, interacting with students online, and upholding academic integrity.
- Information Resource Personnel—identify and locate materials to support content and provide guidance/clearance for the use of copyright materials.
- Mentor/Tutor—assists students and provides general assistance regarding the course organization, either virtually or face-to-face at a remote location.
- Assessor—develops and/or administers student assessments of learning as well as instruments such as course evaluations (p. 14).

It is important to note that some members of the instructional team may assume more than one of the above roles before, during, and after the course development process.

COURSE DEVELOPMENT—TIPS FOR PEDAGOGICAL EFFECTIVENESS

Technology can help create rich learning environments. Many Web-based courses are centered on content delivery and presentation instead of learning. Learning is an ongoing process that is fully optimized when students are actively involved and engaged in the content. One of the most significant impacts of "reconceptualizing" content for Web-delivery is on the teaching style, which empowers instructors to function as facilitators of learning resources, rather than just transmitters of facts and information. Thus, a traditional face-to-face course cannot simply be placed online.

Course content for Web-delivery should be organized into self-contained "manageable chunks" of instruction (e.g., modules or units) and contain an overview of module content, learning objectives/outcomes, Internet resources that support instruction, learning activities, and assessment strategies to account for various learning styles.

Instructional design and multimedia development, as well as innovative curriculum transformation can require a significant investment in time and energy. Table 16.2 (adapted from "Teaching on the Web" at http:// www.lgta. org:8080/design/design.constraint.shtml) illustrates desirable pedagogical methods for developing engaging online learning experiences and the amount of time, expertise, and cost considerations for each.

Effective Web-based research courses incorporate a variety of highly engaging instructional strategies in order to facilitate collaborative approaches to research and opportunities for discussing and disseminating research

Table 16.2 Comparison of Pedagogical Methods

Method	Technology	Engaging	Cost	Time	Expertise
Brainstorming	Forums	High	Free	< 2Days	Can Do Alone
Case Study	Layout, Multimedia	High	Free	< 2 Days	Can Do Alone
Collaborative Learning	Forums	High	Free	< 2 Days	Can Do Alone
Discussions	Forums	Medium	Free	< 2 Days	Can Do Alone
Guest Speakers	Multimedia	High	Moderate (< $2,500)	1 or 2 Weeks	Assistance Needed
Lecture	Text-Based	Low	Free	< 2 Days	Can Do Alone
Lecture (Audio/Video)	Multimedia	Medium	Moderate (< $2,500)	2 or 3 Days	Can Do Alone
Panels	Multimedia	High	Moderate (< $2,500)	< 2 Days	Assistance Needed
Question and Answer	Forums	Medium	Free	< 2 Days	Can Do Alone
Reading	Text-Based	Low	Free	< 2 Days	Can Do Alone
Simulation	Programming, Multimedia	High	Expensive (> $5,000)	1 or 2 Months	Team Approach
Virtual Tours	Layout, Multimedia	High	Moderate (< $2,500)	1 or 2 Weeks	Assistance Needed
Web Quests	Layout, Multimedia	High	Moderate (< $2,500)	1 or 2 Weeks	Assistance Needed

findings. It is important to develop project management plans for the course development process in order to delegate tasks and responsibilities. The entire process of videotaping and digitizing mini-lectures into streaming audio/video format involves the use of video cameras and personal computers equipped for multimedia digital conversion. Another software development tool includes screen capture programs, which create screen shots and record movement displayed on a computer screen, for the purposes of demonstrating the use of a statistical approach (Figure 16.1), selecting value labels, and representing alternate ways of analyzing data.

An alternative approach to developing in-house instructional materials is to browse through the online Multimedia Educational Resource for Learning and Online Teaching (http://www.merlot.org), which is a free collection of Web-based learning objects designed primarily for use in higher education.

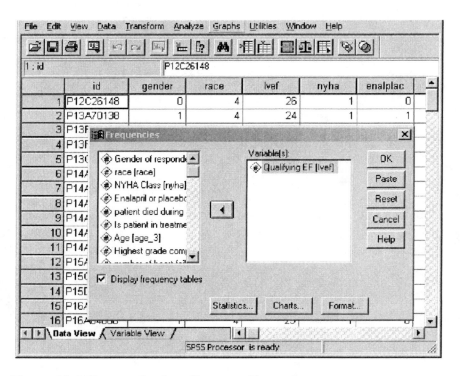

Figure 16.1 Screen Capture Program Example

Copyright/Intellectual Property Issues

There are many underlying copyright and intellectual property issues that need to be considered when developing content and incorporating content into a Web-based course. The Technology, Education, and Copyright Harmonization (TEACH) Act was enacted November 2, 2002 and updated existing U.S. copyright laws to permit the fair use of academic materials for Web-based distance education purposes. The TEACH Act resulted from the U.S. Copyright Office's 1999 Report on Copyright and Digital Distance Education and "amended copyright law to permit professors, under certain circumstances, to use some of the same copyrighted works in online courses that they have used in traditional ones, free of charge and without having to ask permission first" (Carnevale, 2003, p. A29).

Prior to the TEACH Act, copyright laws allowed portions of copyrighted works to be used without permission for instructional purposes, *Fair Use Guidelines for Educational Multimedia* (1996):

- Text material—Up to 10% or 1000 words, whichever is less
- Numerical Data Sets (e.g., databases)—Up to 10% or 2500 fields or cell entries, whichever is less, from a copyrighted database or data table
- Illustrations/Photographs—No more than 5 images from an artist/photographer, or no more than 10% or 15 works from a published collective work
- Motion media (e.g., video)—Up to 10% or 3 minutes, whichever is less

However, one should always review institutional policies and procedures to completely understand fair-use parameters and adhere to specific institutional intellectual property guidelines.

TEACHING/LEARNING STRATEGIES

Strategies for teaching/learning online differ from those employed in the traditional classroom setting. Rather, the challenge to faculty teaching online, especially a research course that requires frequent interaction with and to the ideas and efforts of others, is to build an online learning community that facilitates and enables students to participate and collaborate with each other as they acquire research content and skills.

Interactivity impacts the level of learning that students attain (Vygotsky, 1986), increases cognition (facts, data, mental skills), encourages active engagement in learning (Reeves & Reeves, 1996), and causes students to reflect and articulate ideas (Reeves & Reeves, 1996). Creating online teaching/learning experiences involves three types of interaction:

- Student-Content: Students' interaction with research course content is maximized when: course modules are designed using a variety of engaging instructional strategies, electronic resources, and multimedia learning elements; asynchronous and synchronous communications (discussion boards and chat rooms) are structured around research themes; students are actively engaged in problem-based learning activities that require analysis, synthesis, and evaluation, thus facilitating their achievement of higher levels of critical thinking (Bloom, 1956).
- Student-Instructor: Desirable student-instructor interaction is characterized by: explicit standards for timely feedback regarding course assignments; frequent use of e-mail, discussion boards, and/or chat rooms in a manner that facilitates the attainment of learning objectives; and the incorporation of life experiences, interests and ambitions throughout the interaction.
- Student-Student: Student to student interaction is best achieved when: student participation is required; varied and multiple opportunities are afforded for collaborative group work via e-mail, discussion boards, and chat rooms; and group deliverables e.g.,decisions, plans and designs, proposals, case studies, problem solutions) are clearly defined.

Frequent opportunities for student-content, student-instructor, and student-student interaction are essential for establishing and building a strong online community of learners in a Web-based research course.

COURSE STRUCTURE

A well-designed Web-based research course must account for diverse learning styles and provide strategies that lead to successful engagement in the research process, thus allowing all students the opportunity to master content and to develop research, organizational, and motivational skills. Students do not have to be technologically sophisticated to take a Web-based course, however, they should be familiar with basic computer operations and keyboarding skills (such as opening/saving documents, exploring Web sites, and following directions), have a minimum degree of comfort in using technology, and have access to their own personal computer connected to an internet service provider. Additional technical requirements for audio/video streaming, and accessing password-protected electronic databases and journals must be indicated well in advance before students enroll in a Web-based course. Of particular importance is ensuring that students have access via print, CD-ROM, or online to the Cumulative Index of Nursing Allied Health Literature (CINAHL) database, which is well-known for its large repository of nursing research literature.

Student involvement in the collection and analysis of data is an important component of a graduate level Web-based research course. Thus, access to statistical software programs that provide tools to uncover facts, patterns, and trends for decision-making purposes; display results in graphical format; and enable students to produce and share research results using a variety of reporting methods must be a primary concern. Several statistical software programs are available; the selection of one over the other will depend on several factors including cost and availability. Table 16.3 presents information regarding the advantages and disadvantages of the statistical packages most frequently employed in Web-based research courses.

Table 16.3 Comparison of Statistical Software

Software	Cost	Advantages	Disadvantages
SPSS	Institution License: $5–10,000 Student License: $299	Comprehensive Analysis Tool	PC-Based
WebStat	Free	Web-Based	Moderate Learning Curve
Microsoft Excel	PartofMicrosoft Office Suite	WidelyAvailable	Limited Tools for Error Detection

The selection of a specific software package will depend on the extent to which students are expected to conduct statistical analysis while taking the Web-based research course and the resources readily available to the institution and students, especially as they relate to cost. Course developers also should review statistical software packages taking into account which software packages will best enable students to achieve the research course objectives and desired outcomes, for example, the level of sophistication of the data analysis to be performed.

FACULTY SUPPORT

Faculty support is an ongoing process—during the course development stage, throughout the online course delivery, and upon course completion. The transition from teaching in a traditional face-to-face environment to an online environment requires sufficient time to learn how to manage delivering a Web-based course, interacting with students online and upholding academic integrity. Depending on the size of the instructional team, opportunities should be provided well in advance for either one-on-one, small group, and/or large group training in the technical use of a courseware management system. Additional training should also occur for managing electronic mail (which increases dramatically while teaching a Web-based course), organizing/creating electronic folders for various submitted assignments, adding electronic comments within student research papers, facilitating group projects and discussions online, and using online tools for detecting cheating and plagiarism. Once the delivery of the Web-based course begins, both technical and instructional assistance should be readily available to resolve any questions or problems that faculty may encounter.

Ideally, provisions should be made for new online instructors to be mentored by experienced online instructors, allowing for the exchange of advice, feedback, guidance, and tips. The opportunity to virtually observe each other's Web-based courses (while in progress or archived) can provide meaningful exchanges of online pedagogy experiences.

Due to the increased amount of time expended while developing, delivering, and maintaining a Web-based course, as compared to a traditional course, issues are likely to arise in regard to the need for adjustments in polices/procedures, workload, and/or tenure and promotion criteria. Currently, when such issues arise they are handled in a different manner across institutions and the nature of the adjustments typically is based upon institutional policies, procedures, and usual practices. Thompson (2002) acknowledges consideration of these factors, in terms of compensation and recognition, as demonstrating an institution's commitment to Web-based distance education and directly related to increased faculty satisfaction.

STUDENT SUPPORT

Adequate information regarding the entire online learning experience should be provided to students, so they can determine whether or not Web-based distance education will meet their needs. It is extremely important to anticipate and provide answers to the most frequently asked questions of newcomers to online learning. For example, at the University of Maryland School of Nursing's distance education Web site (http://nursing.umaryland.edu/de/frame.htm), students are able to access admissions and registration material, explore Web-based degree and certificate programs, access previews of Web-based courses, review technical contacts and requirements, download necessary plug-ins, and watch testimonials from experienced online learners.

Once the decision has been made to take a Web-based course, students will expect timely access to Web-based courses at the beginning of the semester and prompt responses from the admissions office, the instructor, and/or the technical support personnel. The instructional team should design and develop specific virtual orientations for each aspect of taking a Web-based course (e.g., logging on for the first time, accessing course materials, and using the communication tools) and arrange traditional face-to-face orientations if geographically feasible, or if not, using interactive video technology. A specific electronic mail account for technical support should be established and provided to all students. In addition, a technical issues and/or a student lounge discussion board within the Web-based research course can provide an opportunity for students to post questions and assist each other with designing research protocols, and collecting, analyzing, and interpreting data. Specific discussion board areas should be set up for students to post and prepare research results, seek peer review of their projects, and discuss/share strategies for gaining institutional review board approval.

A combination of such student support mechanisms will allow faculty to focus on the actual teaching/learning aspect of the Web-based research course instead of addressing a myriad of individual technical questions and strengthen the foundation of the research course's learning community.

EVALUATION AND ASSESSMENT

Evaluation activities should provide for assessment of the various factors in regard to institutional support, course development, teaching/learning, course structure, faculty support, and student support that contribute to the quality of Web-based distance education before and during course implementation and the results should be employed on an ongoing basis for the purpose of continuous quality improvement and/or assurance. For example, factors that characterize a well-designed Web-based research course that should be assessed include clearly stated expectations for course interactivity, appropriate use of technology, and relevant and engaging research assignments.

In addition to determining the extent that students achieve course objectives, national benchmarks and standards employed during course development and implementation should serve as the criteria for determining the quality of course outcomes. For example, student outcomes usually include number of student publications, quality of resulting products such as research protocols, and/or funded projects produced as a result of the learning experience. In settings where both traditional face-to-face and Web-based graduate research courses are offered, it is important to compare such outcomes resulting from each of these approaches.

Multiple methods for data collection from a variety of sources should be employed to gain a comprehensive assessment of all aspects of the course, and the reliability and validity of all data collection methods should be investigated prior to and each time they are used. Course and faculty evaluation instruments and methods employed in the face-to-face traditional research course should be modified to include additional questions relating directly to the online educational experience, and security measures should be taken to ensure the anonymous collection of student information.

EDUCAUSE and Newman (2003, p. 4) recognizes the importance of a comprehensive evaluation of a Web-based course and suggests the possible metrics for measuring the overall online success, as presented in Table 16.4.

Successful Web-based programs should incorporate both student and faculty feedback to promote high interest and satisfaction for all responsible parties involved. Wills and Stommel (2002) note that while student responses are generally favorable to Web-based courses,

Table 16.4 Possible metrics for measuring online success

Category	Data
Institution	• Student Enrollment and Tuition Fee Growth • Market Reach, New Market Opportunities • Improved Classroom Utilization • Alliances and Partnerships
Faculty	• Faculty Awards/Recognition • Technical Competency Improvements • Enhanced Professional Development • Rate/Percentage of Faculty Participation
Students	• Academic Performance • Retention Rates • Course/Program Completion Rates • Salary Increases

pretest/posttest survey results typically highlight the specific needs for adequate socialization and support of students.

In summary, a dedicated technical infrastructure; collaboration among administrators, teaching faculty, and instructional/information technology staff; well-developed project management plans for course development and maintenance; integration of engaging instructional strategies; appropriate support mechanisms for faculty and students; and an ongoing holistic assessment/evaluation process can result in an exciting Web-based graduate research course that encourages digital scholarship and participation in a variety of active learning experiences. Looking toward the future, there are an increasing number of American universities establishing virtual consortiums of Web-based course offerings. This trend is likely to extend internationally, where varying cultural, language, and ethical standards will need to be considered and addressed.

REFERENCES

American Association of Colleges of Nursing. (2003). *Statement on Distance Education Policies.*

Bloom, B.S. (Ed.). (1956). Taxonomy of educational objectives: The classification of educational goals. *Handbook I, Cognitive domain.* New York: Longmans, Green.

Carnevale, D. (2003). Slow start for long-awaited easing of copyright restriction [Electronic version]. *Chronicle of Higher Education, 49*(29), A29.

EDUCAUSE and Newman, A. (2003). Measuring success in Web-based distance learning. *EDUCAUSE Center for Applied Research (ECAR) Research Study.*

Fair Use Guidelines for Educational Multimedia. (1996). Retrieved June 23, 2003, from http://www.loc.gov/copyright/

Institute for Higher Education Policy. (2000). *Quality on the line: Benchmarks for success in Internet-based distance education.* Retrieved June 19, 2003, from http://www.ihep.com/Pubs/PDF/Quality.pdf

Mills, M. E., Fisher, C., & Stair, N. (2001). Web-based courses: More than curriculum. *Nursing & Health Care Perspectives, 22,* 235–239.

Reeves, T., & Reeves, P. (1996). Effective dimensions of interactive learning on the World Wide Web. In B. Kahn (Ed.), *Web-based instruction* (pp. 59–66). Englewood Cliffs, NJ: Educational Technology Publications.

Southern Regional Education Board's Distance Learning Laboratory Faculty Issues Report. (2001). *Supporting faculty in the use of technology: A guide to principles, policies, and implementation strategies* [Electronic version]. Retrieved June 19, 2003, from http://www.electroniccampus.org/policylab/Reports/Supporting_Faculty.pdf

Thompson, M. (2002). Faculty Satisfaction. *Sloan-C View: Perspectives in Quality Online Education, 1*(2), 6. Retrieved June 26, 2003, from http://www.sloan-c.org/publications/view/v1n2/coverv1n2.htm

US Copyright Office's Report on Copyright and Digital Distance Education. (1999). Retrieved June 19, 2003, from http://www.copyright.gov/ reports/de_rprt.pdf

Vygotsky, L. S. (1986). *Thought and language.* Cambridge, MA: Institute of Technology Press.

Wills, C. E., & Stommel, M. (2002). Graduate nursing students' precourse and postcourse perceptions and preferences concerning completely Web-based courses. *Journal of Nursing Education, 41*(5), 9.

Chapter 17

PhD Programs Online

Carol M. Patton, Patricia Fedorka, and Natalie Pavlovich

This chapter highlights curriculum, course management systems, resources, skill development, and methodologies to support online PhD programs in nursing. Internet-based PhD programs provide access to educational content for development of research expertise and continued pursuit of research and scholarship.

Internet-based PhD programs make doctoral eduction available to those students living in remote and rural areas or in other parts of the international community with limited ability to attend doctorial courses in a traditional classroom. An emphasis on creating learning environments that focus on helping students develop and explore ways to attain scholarship and study the science of nursing via the Internet is particularly important.

PHD CURRICULUM: AN EXAMPLE

Many of the earliest online PhD programs were derived from computer-enhanced courses that then were developed into a totally online program. Despite different delivery modes, the established core content remained the same: nursing theory, research and statistical methods, and selected cognates to enhance learning experiences. Students individually collaborate with faculty to develop an individualized study plan to meet individual learning needs.

Course Management System (CMS) for the Duquesne University PhD Program

During the initial years of the PhD program, Duquesne University School of Nursing (DUSON) offered classes via the Internet using a Course Management System called First Class. As of 2003 the CMS system for offering distance education for the PhD students in nursing was Blackboard 5.5. The Blackboard 5.5 CMS platform has allowed nursing faculty to enhance and supplement traditional classroom teaching primarily through faculty roles that include but are not limited to planning, design, implementation, administration, and direct instruction of course materials and content in each of the doctoral courses in the curriculum. It was important for DUSON faculty to find a CMS that facilitated student/faculty needs in terms of user friendliness and would encourage students to develop lifelong scholarship and research trajectories using Internet-based technology. Faculty and the Computer Technical Support Service Department (CTS) discussed available CMS educational platforms. It was particularly important to determine ways an Internet-based curriculum could enhance student learning and lifelong scholarship and research trajectories. Strategies to connect PhD students with expert researchers in their areas of interest and to assist students in discerning the quality of research in their respective areas of interest were important considerations.

Initially the PhD courses were delivered using synchronous chats, usually one evening a week for 3 hours. Faculty philosophy was focused largely on the need to have teaching presence using CMS platforms, to find the best fit for student-faculty engagement in Internet-based classrooms, and to maintain pedagogy/androgogy. It was evident in pioneering the Internet-based PhD curriculum that faculty had to multitask in the classroom to develop and deliver the technology while maintaining curricular rigor and program standards. It also became apparent to faculty teaching in the Internet-based environment that teaching strategies take considerable teacher effort. It was also evident that faculty had to utilize a variety of strategies to engage the learner in an interactive and engaging learning process to assist students to embrace value and appreciation for lifelong learning (Anderson, Rourke, Garrison, & Archer, 2001; Bullen, 1998; Kanuka & Anderson, 1998).

Faculty philosophy was an important consideration in the choice of CMS systems for the PhD nursing program. When the PhD program began, the CMS that seemed consistent with the philosophy of the

DUSON was First Class. This system allowed faculty to post relevant course materials for students and to create pedagogically and andro-gogically rigorous strategies for interactive student learning. Specific pedagogical features of the First Class CMS were the ability to plan, design, facilitate, and evaluate enhancement of cognitive and social processes of PhD students in attaining program goals, primarily to provide meaningful and educationally worthwhile learning outcomes with respect to a scholarly career and research trajectory to move professional nursing forward in the research arena. The PhD curriculum had the right elements and now the challenge was to find the right fit with a CMS that enhanced faculty and student interaction to accomplish program goals.

The major benefits of the First Class CMS were the underpinnings to assist faculty to build courses in the PhD curriculum with emphasis on process, structure, evaluation, and interaction components in each course. CMS-assisted learning afforded faculty the opportunity to have teaching presence in the PhD curriculum and move students toward higher-order thinking. Strategies used included re-purposing already prepared traditional course materials, providing commentary and mini-lectures to students, providing personal insight into theory and research as a curricular thread through all courses in the PhD curriculum, creating variation in groups of students in the virtual classroom with group assignments, and providing online feedback to students that was both accurate and timely. The decision was made to move toward Blackboard because this CMS allowed faculty to customize courses building on the First Class CMS.

Once a CMS is chosen, it is important to have a university department that can provide the infrastructure support and faculty development, and serve as a resource to students entering the virtual educational environment. This department also serves to assist faculty in pedagogical course components and organization of the course in a way that also reflects the visual and interactive dynamics of the Internet to capture and engage students in the learning experience.

Blackboard 5.5 CMS has fostered and promoted creation of a culture of online learners by promoting quick responses either by e-mail or telephone from both students and faculty when working within the CMS. Faculty are able to post assignments and course information, have hotlinks to designated Web sites that enhance course concepts, post discussions between and among student groups as assigned to monitor dialogue and make content corrections as needed, provide timely feedback on course-related matters to students, and test students online with immediate feedback if that option is selected. Blackboard 5.5 allows prompt e-mail communication between students and faculty. It is helpful too for all students to have e-mail access prior to course enrollment. At DUSON, students are required to have a university-based e-mail address. Students may then forward the e-mail to another personal address if they desire. Many times students change e-mail addresses but do not update their address with the school, university, or faculty. This becomes particularly problematic in communicating with students. Mandatory university-based e-mail addresses help to limit some problems and to deliver accurate and timely course-related materials. Students are also informed of CMS system upgrades or important notifications via Blackboard 5.5.

One of the major issues confronting faculty and students in an Internet-based PhD curriculum is system overload during peak class hours when courses are offered synchronously. There often are many courses occurring during peak evening hours. Thus, for example, at DUSON it was not uncommon for the CMS to experience difficulties such as students and faculty getting "bumped off line" during synchronous discussions. As Internet-based courses grew in numbers and participants, so did the infrastructure issues. It was during this time that the decision was made to offer courses exclusively in the asynchronous mode.

Asynchronous delivery method meant necessary upgrades of courses by some faculty depending on original course design and strategies already in place to engage doctoral students in their courses. The first sets of evaluative data are pending with respect to asynchronous approaches to course delivery. An example of using asynchronous methodologies for the research sequence is that students are asked to participate and engage in substantive discussion via the Discussion Board. One example of such an assignment would be to ask students to review the Web site for the Agency for Healthcare Research and Quality (AHRQ) (http://www.ahrq.gov) and determine priority areas for nursing research. Sites like AHRQ assist PhD students to access Internet-based sites to locate those agencies that provide private and federal funding to support nursing research. Students can also use the Internet to do literature searches and find cutting edge technology or methodologies pertinent to their areas of research interest. PhD students can also select top nursing research experts as members of their doctoral committee through interactions via the Internet that they might not otherwise have had available in the traditional classroom and thus benefit from research mentorship from a distance.

ELECTRONIC DISSERTATIONS

Many universities have developed mechanisms for students to submit their dissertations electronically. In some institutions students are required to do so. Major benefits of electronic dissertations are that they: (a) prepare students for publication post graduation by providing training in electronic publication, (b) provide more immediate and wider exposure of students' research, (c) enhance students' presentation and communication skills, and (d) allow students to have a hyperlink to the thesis/dissertation from their home page.

Electronic dissertations are submitted to ProQuest, a private company that formerly was known as the UM Microfilms. Submission requirements for electronic dissertations are provided by an institution's library. In addition, the library may provide special training for graduate students and faculty via workshops to emphasize document formatting, PDF conversion, and electronic dissertation submission requirements.

DEVELOPING STUDENT SKILLS IN
INTERNET-BASED RESEARCH

A major outcome objective of the PhD curriculum is to prepare graduates with the ability and motivation to establish a program of research. Most traditional PhD programs require students to provide a written statement of the applicant's clinical expertise, research interests, and career goals. Students are admitted based on previous ability to succeed in an accredited master's program in nursing. In addition, applicants to PhD programs are required to provide evidence of scholarly work in nursing that is assessed through evaluation of a master's thesis, published articles, or other equivalent scholarly products. When a PhD applicant has met technical admission criteria, faculty review the application for fit with faculty research interests. Similar research interests among students and faculty provide a mutually beneficial relationship for student and faculty and also provide mentorship for students in developing a scholarly research trajectory. Students communicate with faculty and faculty with students via e-mail and telephone communication throughout their program.

EVALUATION OF INTERNET-BASED PHD PROGRAMS

Structure, process, and outcome of any program provide important clues to areas that are successful as well as areas that warrant improvement. The American Association of Colleges of Nursing (AACN) criteria and standards for evaluation are appropriate documents to evaluate online PhD programs. Student and course evaluations should reflect the AACN standards for doctoral education. Students complete evaluations for each course and faculty member at the end of every semester. Student, faculty, and course evaluations for the PhD program reflect student satisfaction with Internet-based PhD programs.

REFERENCES

Anderson, T., Rourke, L., Garrison, D. R., & Archer, W. (2001). Assessing teaching presence in a computer-assisted conferencing context. *Journal of Asynchronous Learning Networks, 5*(2), 1–17.

Bullen, M. (1998). Participation and critical thinking in online university distance education. *Journal of Distance Education, 13*(2), 1–32.

Kanuka, H., & Anderson, T. (1998). Online social interchange, discourse, and knowledge construction. *Journal of Distance Education, 13*(1), 57–74.

Chapter 18

Internet-Based Continuing Education in Research

Kristen S. Montgomery

M any opportunities exist to obtain continuing education for nurses via the Internet. Some of these options include improvements in skills or caring for a specific patient population. Additionally, numerous sites exist where individuals are required to read an article and then complete questions about the article's content to receive continuing education on a variety of topics. In recent years, as there has been an increased focus on the care nurses provide and the outcomes of nursing care, an emphasis has been placed on evidence-based nursing practice. Continuing education opportunities exist to receive "updates" on the latest standard of care for a patient population by practicing in a way that is evidence-based. In addition to providing nursing "content" updates, continuing education has begun to focus on research methods. In the future, we can expect to see the area of research continuing education expand further as more programs are developed and more nurses gain the expertise needed to develop Internet-based courses. Of course, the numbers of nurses utilizing any research continuing education offering will drive the existence and growth of them.

The focus of this chapter is identification of specific research continuing education courses that may be useful to nurses who are interested in learning more about research or to more experienced researchers who are looking to develop new research skills or expand existing ones. In addition, the chapter will also address other usages for research continuing education beyond an individual earning continuing education credits for themselves for licensure or certification requirements.

SPECIFIC COURSES OF RESEARCH CONTINUING EDUCATION FOR NURSES

Only one comprehensive continuing education course was identified that focused exclusively on nursing research. This course is titled: "Research Training: Preparing Nurse Scientists" and is sponsored by the National Institute of Nursing Research (NINR). The Web address is: http://www.nih.gov/ninr/news-info/nurse_scientists.html. This course is the online version of the 3 1/2 day course that was previously offered at the National Institutes of Health (NIH). The content of the course is geared toward nurse scientists who have never been PIs of an NIH research project. The course covers the NIH, grantsmanship, and practical skills for advancing a scientific career. Learning objectives are presented at the beginning of the course and include:

- Discuss the general profile of NINR including its organizational structure, mission, strategic plan, research and training opportunities, and impact.
- Discuss the general profile of the Clinical Center including the research and training opportunities it provides and the role of nurses in the intramural research projects.
- Describe key funding mechanisms used by NIH.
- Articulate the four elements necessary for developing a competitive application.
- Articulate strategies for developing a competitive application for research development awards.
- Describe the process in which a grant proposal is received, referred, and goes through peer review at NIH.
- Recognize the review criteria adopted in the scientific review process.
- Recognize the assistance provided by NINR program directors and grants management throughout the grant application process.
- Derive strategies for developing a successful research program from the perspectives of new researchers, seasoned researchers, and nursing school deans.

- Recognize issues related to ethical conduct of research.
- Recognize key IRB principles.
- Discuss research dissemination in terms of organization techniques, submitting abstracts and manuscripts, and evaluating self-progress.
- Identify common issues in recruiting and retaining diverse populations for research.

A registration form must be completed to take the course and for processing of contact hours. The course is presented in 5 sequential modules. The Web page includes a course orientation and a fully moderated message board. Content for the course may be supplemented with videotapes that are available for purchase through the Web site. Completion of the course provides 5 contact hours of continuing education through the Maryland Nurses Association. While there is a cost associated with purchase of the videotapes, the online portion of the course is free.

While the NINR "Research Training: Preparing Nurse Scientists" course is the only research-focused continuing education (CE) that was identified, other sites are available that provide CE based on published research articles. One such site is www.nurselearning.com. Other sites also feature this type of continuing education and can be located on the World Wide Web by searching for "nursing research continuing education."

For those individuals who wish to create continuing education courses, there are opportunities for grant funding via the National Institute of Child Health and Human Development (NICHHD) through the continuing education training grant (T15). This grant mechanism is designed to assist institutions to establish, expand, or improve programs of continuing professional education, especially for programs dealing with new developments in the science or technology of the profession. According to the Web site, the mechanism is intended for the support of short, advanced-level courses (a few days to a few weeks) to emphasize new technologies and enhance skills of scientists. Information on this grant mechanism can be found at: http://www.nichd.nih.gov/training/training_grant.htm.

The Internet can also be useful for identifying courses that are held at a specific location in classroom format or on paper. Research CE opportunities exist in other institutes at NIH. The National Human Genome Research Institute (NHGRI) at: www.genome.gov and the

National Institute of Aging (NIA) at www.nia.nih.gov are examples. The NIH also has a "research and training opportunities" site that is available at: www.training.nih.gov. This link includes tenure track opportunities, student opportunities, fellowships, and CE for psychologists and physicians.

THE ROLE OF RESEARCH CONTINUING EDUCATION IN THE BROADER CONTEXT OF NURSING

Internet-based research CE is useful for individuals who wish to develop additional expertise and skills related to various aspects of the research process. In addition to the use of online research CE by individuals, other useful applications exist. For example, research continuing education can be useful to supplement traditional research courses or can be used as a component of distance education courses. In-depth courses such as that offered by NINR are ideal as they offer comprehensive content. The federal compliance course on the ethical use of subjects in human research (available at: http://cme.cancer.gov/c01) is another example of research continuing education that may be useful for research courses. The National Cancer Institute in collaboration with several other NIH institutes developed this course. Any individuals who are conducting research with human subjects must prove that they have training in research ethics; thus, this type of continuing education can offer convenience for busy faculty and graduate students who may have difficulty integrating a paper-and-pencil course into their busy schedules. Online research continuing education can be completed any place that one can access the Internet, 24 hours a day. Please see the chapters in this text on undergraduate and graduate education for additional information.

Research courses that are offered online can also be useful in training research assistants (RAs) who will work on various projects. In addition to research ethics training, RAs will need to understand and appreciate the complexities involved in Internet-based research. Research ethics training online for a project will also meet the student's requirement for his or her own research projects (e.g., a thesis or dissertation). In some instances a student may be able to earn independent study credits for in-depth courses.

SUMMARY

Many continuing education opportunities exist via the Internet; some offerings focus on research findings and, increasingly, research methods. NINR offers a comprehensive research course that is of high quality and may be useful for new researchers and in a variety of educational offerings in nontraditional formats (e.g., online courses, distance education). It is likely that continuing education offerings that focus on research will continue to increase in numbers.

Chapter 19

Challenges in Research Utilization for Educators and Clinicians

Meredith Wallace

The progression of nursing science has been fostered by research in nursing and other disciplines for the past century. However, it is evident that for the research to be valuable for patient care and for the science of nursing to progress further, research must be utilized. Models of evidence-based nursing are currently taught in all levels of nursing education. However, in any nursing research class within which the importance of nursing research has been clearly integrated, undergraduate, RN students completing BSN degrees, and graduate students can identify examples of outdated clinical practice that are not reflective of currently available nursing research. It is important for faculty teaching undergraduate nursing courses, including both clinical and research courses, to integrate the latest nursing and health care research into the courses.

Effective utilization of nursing research relies on many factors, which have been conceptualized into research utilization models (CURN, 1983; Donaldson, 1992; Bostrom & Wise, 1994; Rosswurm & Larrabee, 1999). Regardless of the model used to guide the integration of research into practice, most researchers agree that the first step requires nurses to question current practice. This assumes that nurses value and understand nursing research and its role in changing practice. Many clinicians would be at a loss to provide the scientific rationale behind many common nursing practices, such as application of restraints to keep older adults from falling. The response to why this commonly used practice is being done would likely be "because we have always done it." This example clearly underscores the need for a consistent integration of research within all academic nursing courses.

Effective research utilization also requires access to the research. Cronenwett (1995) reported that effective methods of disseminating nursing research included conferences and print materials. Accessing information is the phase in which the Internet is most useful. The availability of the Internet to gather clinical information has removed a major barrier to research utilization. However, easy access to good information is also easy access to bad information. Nurses must become educated consumers of nursing research to know which information is ready to be integrated into nursing practice and which is not.

Finally, successful integration of nursing research into practice requires removal of institutional barriers. Organizational character-istics identified as barriers to research utilization include both avail-able facilities and cooperation of staff. It is only when nurses acknowl-edge that practice needs to change, access appropriate knowledge to make that change, and can successfully change practice, that evi-dence-based practice occurs.

Little information is available to guide the utilization of nursing research with the use of the Internet. A Cumulative Index to Nursing and Allied Health Literature (CINAHL) search using the words "research utilization and the Internet" revealed only seven articles. Of these resources, two were found not to be applicable to the current topic. Three were research-based articles and two were review articles.

Montgomery, et al. (2001) presented a model for ideal utilization of nursing research on an international level, through partnerships between investigators and clinicians. However, the reality is that such models are rarely implemented. With the emergence of the Internet to aid in access to research, there is no time like the present to begin to form these partnerships and develop evidence-based practice envi-ronments internationally. Their article begins by reviewing the barri-ers to research utilization. One of these includes the small amount of multi-lingual nursing research that is culturally congruent and avail-able in countries other than the United States. Other barriers include limited knowledge and support for research utilization. While the Inter-net presents a theoretical alternative to overcoming some of these barriers, availability and limited knowledge of its use continues to be an obstacle. Despite these continuing barriers, the authors reported that advances in research dissemination are occurring. Specifically, the researchers listed goals of the International Council of Nurses (ICN) toward overcoming these barriers and also the introduction of Internet-based research reviews in undergraduate and graduate nursing programs and global collaborations to foster research utilization at an international level (Montgomery, et al.).

Logan reported in 2001 that consumers use Medline more than nurses. She contended that nurses may be left behind in their knowledge about clinical issues and underscores the need for them to be knowledgeable about up-to-date clinical research information via the Internet. Her article focused on the introduction of Internet literature searches during undergraduate nursing education and provided practical information on how this can be accomplished. As with much of the information available on research utilization, evaluation of research findings for clinical practice with a specific focus on the critical appraisal of Internet information was discussed. During this discussion, the author focused the critique on the origin of the Internet information as a major determinant in evaluating its usefulness for clinical practice. The author also challenged nurses to teach patients how to effectively utilize the Internet to gain credible health information.

Two articles were focused on the utilization of research to foster a particular specialization in nursing. Watkins, Mills and Gillibrand (2001) reported on an ongoing collaboration project between nurses specializing in diabetes and an academic center in England. Using the Internet, information was gathered to foster improved clinical practice with effectiveness. Ciliska, Hayward, Dobbins, Brunton, and Underwood (1999) conducted a study to determine the barriers to research utilization of public health decision makers. The sample included 242 respondents of whom 80–92% reported that lack of time, availability of research results and resources to implement research were moderate to very serious barriers to research utilization. This study did not focus on the utilization of research by nurses, nor did it specifically address the use of the Internet for nursing research utilization.

A report by Royle, Blythe, DiCenso, Baumann, and Fitzgerald (1997) discussed a study of 67 vice-presidents and directors of nursing to determine the resources, organizational structures, and training needs of nurses to facilitate research utilization. The results showed that all hospitals had libraries, but some of the smaller ones did not have electronic access to research. Of all respondents, 69% were interested in acquiring these databases and 62% believed training in the use of Internet-based literature searches was needed.

Little information is available to guide the use of the Internet in research utilization. The literature shows that while some provider facilities and institutions are certainly better than others, barriers to the effective integration of research into clinical practice are a prevalent and common theme. Further research on the effective use of the Internet to enhance research utilization is essential to foster evidence-based practice environments.

ASKING THE QUESTION

Goode (1995) reported that the first step to research utilization is identifying a clinical problem or realizing that there may be new information available which leads nurses to question current clinical practice. However, early work by Tierney (1987) and later supported by Cronenwett (1995) purported that exposure to essential new knowledge may occur without asking the question. In general, for nurses to effectively utilize nursing research, they have to identify that new information is available and value the role of that information in changing practice. This requirement presents the first barrier to research utilization; in order for it be overcome, the nurse must acknowledge that the way things are done is not always necessarily the right way.

Closs and Cheater (1994) suggested that both interest and education are essential to change attitudes toward the role of research in clinical practice. Currently practicing nurses may not have had a research course and may find the whole subject intimidating. However, new interest in research may be stimulated by reading information that may be immediately applicable to improving practice. To generate an interest and appreciation for research among nurses, it is essential that nurses be aware that new pieces of evidence are currently being used clinically.

Once nurses become aware that research is being used, at least to some extent in their setting, it may be helpful to decide upon a prevalent problem and then, with the assistance of a more experienced research clinician, conduct an Internet review of the literature to see what information is available. This can be accomplished on a one-on-one basis, with the nurses and a research mentor, or in an in-service or continuing education program. Liaisons between clinical agencies and academic environments are one way to connect researchers with clinicians (Funk, Tornquist, & Champagne, 1995). The researchers report on the Western Interstate Commission for Higher Education (WICHE) program, which provided a model in which nurse educators and clinical nurses are paired for a number of educational workshops to identify clinical problems and strategies for change. It is important, however, that the problems identified come from the nurses, in order for them to realize the utility of the research to them. If something saves nurses time and improves patient outcomes, nurses are likely to use it. Attendance at professional nursing conferences, in which research information is shared, is an excellent way of generating interest, improving attitudes, and raising levels of excitement among practicing nurses.

Interest and education about research is now available in all baccalaureate nursing programs. Phillips (1986) proposed that the most important objective in educating nurses about research is improving appreciation and enthusiasm for utilization of research in the clinical setting. Students must be engaged in seeking solutions to clinical problems they have experienced throughout their baccalaureate curriculums, not just in one research course. When possible, students should be actively involved in faculty research at all educational levels. Only then will they be comfortable solving these problems after graduation.

OBTAINING THE INFORMATION

The availability of the Internet on nursing units in acute-care facilities and laptops with wireless access for homecare nurses has removed a major barrier to utilization of nursing research across these settings. Closs and Cheater (1994) reported that, while access to information may have improved, literature retrieval skills and time may not have. Furthermore, Rosswurm and Larrabee (1999) reported that nurses continue to have trouble understanding the Internet-acquired evidence and integrating it at a sufficient level to change practice. Cronenwett (1995) indicated that language and the methods of conducting and analyzing research are unfamiliar to many practicing nurses, who may or may not have had a course in nursing research. She further listed lack of time as a barrier to understanding the research and integrating it into practice.

The inability of nurses to understand nursing research may lead to the use of publicly available search engines to answer clinical questions. Search engines such as Lycos, Dogpile, Yahoo, etc. are readily available on the Internet and nurses are likely to be familiar with them. However, these publicly available search engines are limited in their ability to provide current research. For example, suppose a nurse cares for a 78-year-old man who presents himself to the emergency department with an inability to urinate for the past 24 hours. Considering the possibility of urethral obstruction by an enlarged prostate gland in this patient, she examines the blood work for a prostate specific antigen (PSA), but finds it close to normal. In seeking another source of the obstruction, she reviews all the patient's prescription and non-prescription medications. She finds that the patient is taking an herbal supplement known as Saw-Palmetto and decides to use a popular search engine to find out more information on this medication. Her search leads to a variety of nutraceutical websites that advertise Saw-Palmetto as an essential component of prostate health, but nothing is found linking this to the previously theorized obstruction—other than the fact that the patient was trying to prevent a prostate problem.

One way to optimize popular search engines to find research-based patient information is to use some of the newer available guides, such as *Internet Resources for Nurses* (Fitzpatrick & Montgomery, 2002) and *Nurses' Guide to Consumer Health Web Sites* (Fitzpatrick, Romano, & Chasek, 2001). Guides such as this have utilized expert nurse authors to identify the best Web sites on a given clinical topic of interest. In absence of such a guide, government Web sites, such as the National Institutes of Health (http://www.nih.gov) or the Centers for Disease Control (http://www.cdc.gov), are easy to remember and better alternatives than popular search engines.

However, while some Web sites are more research-based than others, evidence-based practice relies on direct sources of nursing research. The most popular sources for this literature are the Cumulative Index to Nursing and Allied Health Literature (CINAHL) and MEDLINE or PubMed. Using the patient example from above, the knowledgeable nurse may enter the term "saw-palmetto" in CINAHL and find several articles linking this nutraceutical to artificially low PSA levels in prostate disease patients. Conn et al. (2003) stated that while CINAHL and MEDLINE are "excellent starting points" nurses may miss rigorous studies using new interventions with non-significant findings and small samples. These authors suggested expanding literature searches to include many Internet-based databases and searches of ancestries, citation indexes, research registries, and other available research databases. Unfortunately, most Internet research databases are not publicly available Web sites. Access to the information contained in these databases requires both membership and payment on an individual or institutional level. It is essential that nurses have access to these Internet-based databases to obtain the best information to guide evidence-based practice.

Regardless of the Web site used to access information, a short course in computer-based literature searches and Boolean logic is necessary. Boolean logic is essential in order to gain the search skills needed to gather the most appropriate information for a given inquiry. Boolean logic involves the use of words and symbols within search engines to refine the search. Information on Boolean logic is available at most libraries and it is very helpful in searching for the right information.

The critical appraisal of available research is an essential step toward evidence-based practice. Trammer, Kisilevsky and Muir (1995) conducted a research utilization study with Neonatal Intensive Care Unit (NICU) nurses, consisting of four 2-hour workshops on critiquing the literature. The intervention used group practice to critique two research studies, using a critiquing guide and individual synthesis of the findings. Critiquing skills increased significantly ($t = 2.9$, $p < 0.01$) for eight of the nine group participants. This study is important because it showed that in a brief 8 hours, this major barrier to research utilization may be overcome. In fact, with the great availability of research critiquing guides (Ryan, 1996) and a nurse-researcher or educator, these types of workshops may be created in any practice environment. Follow-up studies are needed to address how long nurses may retain the knowledge learned during the intervention.

A further step needed to change practice is a synthesis of the available research on the topic. Apart from the availability of meta-analyses, one research article on a topic rarely provides the impetus for practice change. It is necessary for nurses to critically review all relevant literature on a topic and present a synthesis of the findings in order to begin to integrate the Internet-acquired evidence into practice. It is important to note that while many acute-care and homecare agencies provide access to the Internet for nursing research, many others do not. Access to the Internet on units of long-term care facilities is rare and many rural hospitals and community providers are not yet "online." For these providers, nurses must continue to rely on their own computers, nursing journals, and conferences to gather Internet-acquired evidence to support and change practice. While efforts should continue to be made to support these alternate forms of knowledge acquisition, computer-based information retrieval does not appear to be a passing trend. In addition, more and more Internet journals, search engines, and information sources are appearing each day. It is essential that nurses be provided access to workplace Internet access for evidence-based practice to be implemented.

ADMINISTRATIVE EMBRACE

Rosswurm and Larrabee (1999) reported evidence-based practice is most likely to be found in clinical areas in which it is valued. However, in this busy clinical environment, it is often difficult for administration to value the role of research in improving practice. Consequently, the infrastructure necessary for practice to be questioned and new answers found is absent in many clinical settings. This occurs despite the great deal of knowledge available supporting the positive outcomes of research utilization on both nurses, job satisfaction and patient care. Trammer, Kisilevsky, and Muir (1995) stated that "when jobs are enriched with research and clinical knowledge, traditional roles can be expanded and nurses' work becomes more satisfying" (p. 27).

Rutledge and Donaldson (1995) reported that organizational components necessary for evidence-based practice must stem from the mission, philosophy, and goals of an institution and then be operationalized within role performance expectations, strategic responsibilities and resources, and the effective evaluation of research utilization. In a research project developed to test this model, researchers found that 65% of the nursing units involved reported becoming "more research oriented" (p. 14). In some institutions, the mission, philosophy, and goals clearly reflect evidence-based practice and they are operationally functioning toward accomplishing these. In others, there is a disconnect between the primary components and their operation. In still others, the mission, philosophy, and goals need updating to reflect evidence-based practice.

It is essential that nursing administration develop a research capacity within a clinical environment. Such an environment allows the free questioning of existing nursing practice and an openness to new approaches to nursing care. It would be rich in journal clubs, research committees, and research presentations, as well as support and opportunities to participate in these activities outside the workplace. Funk, Tornquist, and Champagne (1995) issued a call for nurse administrators to act as role models by participating in research activities and expecting their nurses to do the same. The formalization of this expectation should be found in the nurse's role description and performance appraisal, in order for it to change from something "nice to do" to something that must be done.

Funk, Tornquist, and Champagne (1995) also reported that improved access to research and assistance with understanding it are key desires of nurses seeking evidence-based practice environments.

Nurse administrators must create an environment where as many Internet-based research databases as possible are readily available to the bedside nurse. This may entail upgrading computers, strategically positioning computers for easy access, and removing password barriers. Small grants from local groups or pharmaceutical companies may help with this administrative change. Partnerships between clinicians, researchers, and administrators are essential to allow the utmost availability of professionals who are appreciative and knowledgeable about clinical problems, information seeking, and integration, to infiltrate the clinical area (Funk, Champagne, Tornquist & Weise, 1995).

When practice has been questioned, new strategies sought and synthesized, and a plan for change developed, the administrative embrace calls for nurse researchers to create an environment of change. A study by Funk, Champagne, Tornquist, and Weise (1995) found that 45% of the sample reported that the inability of administration to allow implementation of research was a great or moderate barrier to evidence-based practice. Regardless of how effectively the problem has been articulated and the literature searched and synthesized, change presents risk and is associated with fear of the unknown. However, regardless of the risk, change must be allowed to happen for evidence-based practice to be established. Finally, no discussion about administrative support toward evidence-based practice can be complete without the appeal for adequate staffing so nurses have the time and energy to question, search, and integrate research into practice.

In summary, the successful integration of currently available research into clinical areas is essential to create an environment of evidence-based practice. However, the literature shows that many barriers remain to creating evidence-based practice environments. The emergence of the Internet has been extremely influential in eliminating these barriers. The following tips, adapted from Closs and Cheater (1994), may be helpful in using the Internet to enhance research utilization in the clinical setting.

- Develop a climate of opinion in which research is valued and appreciated as an integral part of clinical practice.
- Generate an interest and appreciation for research among nurses and demonstrate how one or two newer pieces of evidence are currently being used clinically. Then decide upon a prevalent

problem and together review the literature, decide on a practice plan, and implement it. If something saves nurses time and improves patient outcomes, nurses are likely to use it.

• Create a system in which nurses are paired with nurse researchers or educators to develop search and appraisal and synthesis skills.

• Create an environment where as many Internet-based research databases as possible are readily available to the nurse. This may entail upgrading computers, strategically positioning computers for easy access, and removing password barriers.

• From an institutional standpoint, require and reward evidence searches and utilization with certificates, promotions, and acknowledgment.

REFERENCES

Bostrom, J., & Wise, L. (1994). Closing the gap between research and practice. *Journal of Nursing Administration, 24*(5), 22–27.

Ciliska, D., Hayward, S., Dobbins, M., Brunton, G., & Underwood, J. (1999). Transferring public-health nursing research to health-system planning: Assessing the relevance and accessibility of systematic reviews. *Canadian Journal of Nursing Research, 31,* 23–36.

Closs, S. J., & Cheater, F. M. (1994). Utilization of nursing research: Culture, interest and support. *Journal of Advanced Nursing, 19,* 762–773.

Conn, V. S., Isaramali, S., Rath, S., Jantarakupt, J., Wadhawan, R., & Dash, Y. (2003). Beyond MEDLINE for literature searches. *Journal of Nursing Scholarship, 35,* 177–182.

Conduct and Utilization of Research in Nursing Project (CURN). (1983). Using research to improve nursing practice. *Michigan Nurses Association.* Lansing, MI: Grune & Stratton.

Cronenwett, L. R. (1995). Effective methods for disseminating research findings to nurses in practice. *Nursing Clinics of North America, 30,* 429–438.

Donaldson, N. E. (1992). The OCRUN Oration. *The Newsletter of the Orange County Research Utilization in Nursing Project.*

Fitzpatrick, J. J., & Montgomery, K. S. (2002). *Internet resources for nurses.* (2nd ed.). New York: Springer Publishing.

Fitzpatrick, J. J., Romano, C., & Chasek, R. (2001). *Nurses' guide to consumer health websites.* New York: Springer Publishing.

Funk, S. G., Champagne, M. T., Tornquist, E. M., & Weise, R. A. (1995). Administrators' views on barriers to research utilization. *Applied Nursing Research, 8,* 44–49.

Funk, S. G., Tornquist, E. M., & Champagne, M. T. (1995). Barriers and facilitators of research utilization. *Nursing Clinics of North America, 30,* 395–405.

Goode, C. (1995). Evaluation of research-based nursing practice. *Nursing Clinics of North America, 30,* 421–427.

Logan, M. (2001). Academic education: Fostering use of the Internet for research of clinical issues. *Critical Care Nurse, 21*(6), 30–32.

Montgomery, K. S., Eddy, N. L., Jackson, E., Nelson, E., Reed, K., Stark, T. L., et al.(2001). Global research dissemination and utilization: Recommendations for nurses and nurse educators. *Nursing and Health Care Perspectives, 22,* 124–129.

Phillips, L. R. F. (1986). *A clinician's guide to the critique and utilization of nursing research.* Norwalk, CT: Appleton-Century-Crofts.

Rosswurm, M. A., & Larrabee, J. H. (1999). A model for change to evidence-based practice. *Image: Journal of Nursing Scholarship, 31,* 317–322.

Royle, J. A., Blythe, J., DiCenso, A., Baumann, A., & Fitzgerald, D. (1997). Do nurses have the information resources and skills for research utilization? *Canadian Journal of Nursing Administration, 10*(3), 9–30.

Ryan, M. (1996). Reading and utilizing quantitative nursing research: A guide for the neophyte. *Journal of the New York State Nurses Association, 27*(3), 21–23.

Rutledge, D. N., & Donaldson, N. E. (1995). Building organizational capacity to engage in research utilization. *Journal of Nursing Administration, 25*(10), 12–16.

Tierney, A. J. (1987). Research issues: Putting research to good use. *Senior Nurse, 6,* 10.

Trammer, J. E., Kisilevsky, B. S., & Muir, D. W. (1995). A nursing research utilization strategy for staff nurses in the acute care setting. *Journal of Nursing Administration, 25*(4), 21–29.

Watkins, G., Mills, L., & Gillibrand, W. (2001). An interactive web-based network for diabetes nursing research. *Journal of Diabetes Nursing, 5*(3), 88–92.

Appendix 1

Samples of Internet-Based Research Projects

Survey Research

Kristen S. Montgomery and Julie Heringhausen

As access to the World Wide Web continues to expand, nurse researchers are increasingly conducting survey research via the Internet. Historically, nurse researchers have conducted surveys through mail, telephone, and face-to-face interviews in various settings, including in hospitals, clinics, classrooms, and after workshops. Expansion of surveys to the Internet through Web pages or download increases the diversity of research conducted by nurses and others, and accesses population that may be hard to reach using traditional methods. In this section we highlight some of the survey research that has been done by nurses and other health professionals.

There is a plethora of published survey research on whether or not various groups use the Internet in either their personal or professional lives or to access certain types of information (e.g., current practice standards, information about a certain medical condition). In addition to surveys about Internet use in daily life, numerous surveys have been conducted via the Internet. Selected significant articles are presented here. Since the number of nursing research projects conducting surveys is still very limited, the samples described below include research conducted by other medical professionals as well.

1. SURVEYS OF HEALTH CARE PROVIDERS AND FACULTY

Schellhammer (2003) assessed experience and self-estimation of CPR and cardiac defibrillation skills among a group of 650 German-speaking radiologists. The survey was distributed via e-mail and responses were to be returned via e-mail within a 2-month period. Only 12.6% of the sample responded; those who responded did show an interest in basic and advanced life support and supported regular content updates to keep knowledge current.

Horiguchi et al. (2003) assessed physicians working in child neurology for burnout and general health status. Surveys were returned via the Internet from physicians working in various countries. Twenty-nine responses were analyzed, and compared to a previous study that was isolated to Japan, physicians in this study had poorer mental health. Eight (27.5%) responded that they were burned out, and twenty-seven (93%) had neurotic conditions (Horiguchi et al.). Respondents in this survey did have more positive styles for coping with stress, however.

Christianson, Tiene, and Luft (2002) examined faculty perspectives of teaching undergraduate nursing courses completely online. One hundred seventy-one faculty members completed the online survey. Eighty percent indicated that they spent more time on course development and implementation compared to traditional classroom courses. Forty-seven percent preferred online teaching and described the experience as very successful.

2. SURVEYS FOR SOFTWARE DEVELOPMENT

Wells et al. (2003) conducted a technology survey of nursing programs in the U. S. to determine the predominant operating systems in use in preparation for development of electronic end-of-life teaching tools. The authors found almost universal use of the Microsoft Windows-based computer system with the Microsoft Office Suite software. Netscape and Internet Explorer were the most frequently used Web browsers. Nurse educator respondents to this online survey preferred simple and easy-to-use teaching tools provided via CD-ROM or the Internet.

Im and Chee (2003) conducted a survey of self-identified expert oncology nurses from 10 different countries to develop an initial version of computer software to assist nurses with decision-making about cancer pain reported by women from diverse cultural groups. These data were collected via an Internet-based survey and through e-mail group discussions. Ethnicity, gender, geographical location, and age were all contributors to differences in cancer pain descriptions according to the experts who participated (Im & Chee). Participant comments were used by the investigators to develop a decision-support computer program for cancer pain management.

3. SURVEYS OF WEB SITES OR GROUPS

Martin-Facklam, Kostrzewa, Schubert, Gasse, and Haefeli (2002) evaluated Web sites about St. John's wort for quality of content and adherence to published standards for health information appearing on the Internet. The authors used a cross-sectional survey of 208 randomly chosen sites and found that the content quality of the sites was generally poor and that individuals using the Internet to obtain information about St. John's wort should use sites that are noncommercial in nature and that reference published scientific information (Martin-Facklam, et al.).

Houston, Cooper, and Ford (2002) described characteristics of users of Internet-based depression support groups and assessed whether the use of such groups and the amount of use predicted a change in depression symptoms among 103 individuals recruited into the study from the online support groups. Users had a median age of 40 years, 78.6% were women, and 56.3% were unmarried. Eighty-six percent were currently depressed and over 50% of participants heavily used the support group (defined as 5 or more hours in 2 weeks). Thirty-eight percent preferred online communication to face-to-face counseling with a professional. The authors found that heavy users of the support group were more likely to have resolution of depression during follow-up at 6 and 12 months compared to those who used the support group less.

4. SURVEYS COMPARING THE WEB AND OTHER SURVEY MODALITIES

McCabe, Boyd, Couper, Crawford, and D'Arcy (2002) compared methods of collecting alcohol and other drug-related information via traditional postal mail surveys and a Web-based survey method administered to undergraduate students attending a large Midwestern university. The sample of 7,000 was randomly assigned to the mail mode ($n = 3,500$) or the Web-based mode ($n = 3,500$). The authors found that the Web-based mode had a significantly higher response rate and the final sample better represented the target population in terms of gender mix.

Andersson, Lindvall, Hursti, and Carlbring (2002) conducted a study to describe the prevalence and characteristics of hyperacusis, an unusual intolerance of environmental noise. Survey data was collected via postal mail and the Internet. Five hundred eighty-nine responded to the postal survey (59.7% response rate) and 595 responded to an Internet advertisement for the study (51.9% response rate). The authors found that 9% of the Internet group and 8% of the postal group experienced hyperacusis. Exclusion of participants with hearing impairments resulted in a prevalence of 7.7% and 5.9%, respectively. Hyperacusis was associated with concentration difficulties, use of ear protection, avoidance, tension, and sensitivity to light and colors. No differences were noted among the two data collection strategies.

5. SURVEYS IN TRADITIONAL CLINICAL RESEARCH

Web-based surveys have also been used as the only data gathering mechanism in a variety of different clinical studies that focused on diverse topics. **Cella et al. (2003)** administered the Functional Assessment of Cancer Therapy- Anemia (FACT-An) quality of life instrument to a nationally representative sample of 1,400 individuals via the Internet. These responses were compared to measures taken from a group of individuals who were participating in a clinical trial evaluating epoetin alfa versus placebo in anemic cancer patients. The authors found that the tool displayed good psychometric properties and was able to discriminate between respondents with a history of medical illnesses, including cancer and anemia, and those without (Cella, et al.).

Murray and Fox (2002) examined the relationship between prosthesis satisfaction and body image in a group of 44 lower-limb prosthesis users. Individuals responded to a survey via the Internet. The authors found moderate to high negative correlations between body-image disturbance and prosthesis satisfaction, which were consistent across both genders. Positive correlations were found between prosthesis satisfaction and hours of use and negative correlations were found between prosthesis satisfaction and pain experience. The length of time individuals had the prosthesis was unrelated to other variables (Murray & Fox).

Attarian (2002) surveyed rock climbers regarding their self-perceptions of first aid, safety, and rescue skills. Respondents answered survey questions via the World Wide Web over a 15-month period. Two hundred forty-one climbers competed the survey. Most climbers had received
some type of first-aid training, practiced personal safety, and perceived
themselves to be confident in partner- and self-rescue.

Kear (2002) collected anonymous self-report data from a convenience sample of 29 college students who completed a Web-based
survey of risk-taking, depression, social normative beliefs, and smoking resistance self-efficacy on cigarette smoking behavior. From this
data, the researcher recommended antismoking interventions focused
on enhancing refusal skills and delivered to homogenous groups to
reduce cigarette smoking among college students.

REFERENCES

Andersson, G., Lindvall, N., Hursti, T., & Carlbring, P. (2002). Hypersensitivity
to sound (hyperacusis): A prevalence study conducted via the Internet and
post. *International Journal of Audiology, 41*, 545–554.

Attarian, A. (2002). Rock climbers' self-perceptions of first aid, safety, and rescue skills. *Wilderness and Environmental Medicine, 13*, 238–244.

Cella, D., Zagari, M. J., Vandoros, C., Gagnon, D. D., Hurtz, H. J., & Nortier, J.
W. (2003). Epoetin alfa treatment results in clinically significant improvements
in quality of life in anemic cancer patients when referenced to the general
population. *Journal of Clinical Oncology, 21*, 366–373.

Christianson, L., Tiene, D., & Luft, P. (2002). Web-based teaching in undergraduate nursing programs. *Nursing Education, 27*, 276–282.

Horiguchi, T., Kaga, M., Inagaki, M., Uno, A., Lasky, R., & Hecox, K. (2003). An
assessment of the mental health of physicians specializing in the field of
child neurology. *Journal of Pediatric Nursing, 18*, 70–74.

Houston, T. K., Cooper, L. A., & Ford, D. E. (2002). Internet support groups for
depression: A 1-year prospective cohort study. *American Journal of Psychi-
atry, 159*, 2062–2068.

Im, E. O., & Chee, W. (2003). Decision support computer program for cancer
pain management. *Computers, Informatics, & Nursing, 21*, 12–21.

Kear, M. E. (2002). Psychosocial determinants of cigarette smoking among college students. *Journal of Community Health Nursing, 19*, 245–257.

Martin-Facklam, M., Kostrzewa, M., Schubert, F., Gasse, C., & Haefeli, W.
E. (2002). Quality markers of drug information on the Internet: An evaluation of sites about St. John's wort. *American Journal of Medicine, 113*,
740–745.

McCabe, S. E., Boyd, C. J., Couper, M. P., Crawford, S., & D'Arcy, H. (2002). Mode effects for collecting alcohol and other drug use data: Web and U. S. mail. *Journal of Studies in Alcohol, 63,* 755–761.

Murray, C. D., & Fox, J. (2002). Body image and prosthesis satisfaction in the lower limb amputee. *Disability and Rehabilitation, 24,* 925–931.

Schellhammer, F. (2003). Do radiologists want/need training in cardiopulmonary resuscitation? Results of an Internet questionnaire. *Acta Radiology, 44,* 56–58.

Wells, M. J., Wilke, D. J., Brown, M. A., Corless, I. B., Farber, S. J., Judge, M. K. et al. (2003). Technology survey of nursing programs: Implications for electronic end-of-life teaching tool development. *Computers, Informatics, & Nursing, 21,* 29–36.

Internet-Based Intervention Research

Kristen S. Montgomery

Nursing research methods have grown increasingly more sophisticated over the last decade, from descriptive and exploratory research into the development of effective interventions to improve nursing care and patient outcomes. The same evolution is now being seen in Internet-based research. Initial studies examined the prevalence of Internet use by health care providers and patients. The next wave of research was designed to make comparisons among different groups' Internet use. The quality of various types of Web sites also has been examined. For researchers who have been involved in Internet-based research for some time, the science has moved toward the development of interventions. This section is focused on published research in which the Internet is used as an intervention. "The Internet used as an intervention" can be an intervention delivered via the Internet (e.g., nutrition content) or the intervention can include instruction in Internet use to gather information.

1. INTERVENTIONS DELIVERED VIA THE INTERNET

Merion et al. (2003) examined the effects of an Internet-based multimedia intervention on organ donor registration and family notification. Participants were randomly recruited from individuals viewing a specialty Web site. Ten thousand eight hundred forty-four individuals participated. Following the intervention, willing-to-donate scores increased among adults and teens and individuals were more likely to join a donor registry.

Tate, Jackvony, and Wing (2003) compared the effects of an Internet weight-loss program alone versus a program with the addition of behavioral counseling delivered via e-mail for 1 year. Participants ($n =$ 92) in this study were considered to be at risk for type 2 diabetes and had an average body mass index (BMI) of 33. Average age was 48.5 years (*SD* 9.4 years). Participants were randomized to groups and all participants received one face-to-face counseling session, the same core Internet programs, and were instructed to submit weekly weights. Participants in the intervention group also submitted calorie and exercise information and received weekly e-mail behavioral counseling and feedback. At 12 months, the e-counseling group (intervention) lost more weight and had greater decreases in percentages of initial body weight, BMI, and waist circumference.

Baranowski et al. (2003) designed an Internet-based intervention to prevent obesity among 8-year-old African American girls. Thirty-five girls and their parents were randomly assigned to treatment ($n = 19$) or control ($n = 16$) conditions. Girls in the intervention group attended a special 4-week summer day camp and an 8-week home Internet intervention that included the parent. Girls in the control group attended a different 4-week summer day camp followed by a monthly home Internet intervention that did not include components of the Fun, Food, and Fitness Project. After adjusting for body mass index (BMI) at study entry, there were no significant differences in BMI among the intervention and control groups at the end of the 4-week camp or after the full 12-week intervention. The girls in the intervention group did exhibit a trend toward lower BMI, however, less than half of the intervention group logged on to the study Web site, which limited intervention dose. The authors recommended further study to determine what factors might be used to increase use of the Web site.

Frenn et al. (2003) assessed health disparities in middle school students' nutrition and exercise through a 4-session (Internet and video) intervention with a healthy snack and gym labs in urban, low-middle income middle schools. The authors found that the gym lab was beneficial and that fat in the students' diets decreased with each Internet session. Percentage of fat in food was also decreased significantly among Black, White, and Black/Native American girls in the intervention group.

Krishna et al. (2003) examined an Internet-enabled interactive multimedia asthma education program with a group of 228 children (7–17 years) and their caregivers. Participants were randomly assigned to control and intervention groups. Both groups received traditional patient education based on the National Asthma Education and Prevention Program. Intervention group participants received additional self-management education through the Interactive Multimedia Program for Asthma Control and Tracking. The authors found that the intervention group (both children and caregivers) had greater asthma knowledge, decreased asthma symptom days, and decreased emergency room visits and that children used significantly less daily inhaled corticosteriods at visit 3. Asthma knowledge of the children who participated was correlated with fewer urgent physician visits and less use of quick-relief medicines.

Barrera, Glasgow, McKay, Boles, and Feil (2002) conducted a randomized trial of 160 adults with type 2 diabetes who were novice Internet users with a computer and Internet access to one of four conditions: diabetes information only, a personal self-management coach, social support intervention, or a personal self-management coach and the support intervention. Individuals in the two support intervention groups reported significant increases in support on both a diabetes-specific support and a general-support scale.

Winzelberg et al. (2003) evaluated use of an Internet support group for women with primary breast cancer who were randomly assigned to a 12-week Web-based social support group (Bosom Buddies), which was semi-structured, asynchronous, and moderated by a health care professional. The control group received standard care. The authors concluded that Web-based support has the potential to be useful in reducing depression, cancer-related trauma, and stress among women with primary breast cancer.

Clarke et al. (2002) created an Internet-based cognitive therapy self-help program that was designed to be used as a stand-alone intervention for mild to moderate depression or as an adjunct to treatment for more severe depression. Recruitment brochures were mailed to 699 depressed adults in a private, nonprofit health maintenance organization who received treatment for depression and 6,996 nondepressed adults matched for age and gender. Participants consenting to be in the study were randomized to an experimental Web site ($n = 144$) or a no-access control group ($n = 155$). Both groups were able to obtain/continue traditional treatments for depression. At enrollment, most participants were identified as severely depressed using the Center for Epidemiological Studies Depression Scale

(CES-D). Seventy-four percent of subjects completed at least one follow-up at 4, 8, 16, and 32 weeks after enrollment; however, most participants accessed the Web site infrequently.

Lenert et al. (2003) developed an 8-week Web-based course for smoking cessation that included online tools for self-monitoring of behaviors and computer-tailored e-mail timed to enrollees quit efforts. In a study of 49 smokers, the authors found that the participants viewed the Web site an average of 2 times and completed an average of 2 modules (out of 8 total). Thirty-four participants either quit smoking or had a 50% reduction in cigarette use and in a follow-up interview of 26 participants, e-mail and Web components were rated as equally valuable. The authors note the Web technology can be useful as an intervention medium; however, in the current study participants lacked continued interest in the Web content.

Kemper et al. (2002) assessed the impact of an Internet-based curriculum on health professionals' knowledge, confidence, and clinical practices related to herbs and dietary supplements. Physicians, pharmacists, advanced practice nurses, and dieticians were invited to participate via e-mail and those who chose to participate were randomly assigned to immediate intervention or wait list. Five hundred thirty-seven participated in a 10-week curriculum that consisted of 20 case-based modules, links to reliable Internet resources for additional information, and a moderated listserv discussion group. Baseline scores on knowledge, confidence, and communication were similar and after the first follow-up improvements were seen in all three among the intervention group. At the completion of the course (wait list and intervention groups) scores for both groups were significantly better than at baseline.

2. INTERVENTIONS THAT TEACH INTERNET USE

Kronick et al. (2003) assessed the change in frequency and methods with which a group of rural physicians consulted online medical resources before and after an educational intervention on using the Internet. Physicians were randomly assigned to treatment and control groups and completed surveys before and 3 months after the intervention. The intervention included a 3-hour training session on using the World Wide Web to research patient-related questions. At the 3-month follow-up, the intervention group showed significant improvement in the frequency of Internet use for patient questions, comfort using an online database, and frequency of database use, when compared to the control group.

Edgar, Greenberg, and Remmer (2002) developed Internet lessons for oncology patients and their families. This was a joint project between the hospital volunteer oncology support service and the health services library. Twenty-eight individuals participated in the intervention, which included a one-to-one teaching session with a medical library where participants learned to access Internet sites and locate information specific to their needs. Sessions were well received and at 2 months following the intervention participants attributed their well-being at least partly to the intervention.

3. INTERVENTIONS THAT PROVIDE INTERNET ACCESS

White et al. (2002) conducted a randomized controlled trial to assess the psychosocial impact of providing Internet access to older adults over a 5-month period of time. One hundred individuals from 4 congregate housing sites and 2 nursing facilities were randomly assigned to Internet training or a wait-list control group. The intervention consisted of 9 hours of small group training in 6 sessions over 2 weeks. Computers were available to participants for the next 5 months and the trainer was available 2 hours a week to answer questions. At study completion, 60% of the intervention group continued to use the Internet on a weekly basis. While not significant, there was a trend toward less loneliness and depression among the older adults.

REFERENCES

Baranowski, T., Baranowski, J. C., Cullen, K. W., Thompson, D. I., Nicklas, T., Zakeri, I. E., et al. (2003). The Fun, Food, and Fitness Project (FFFP): The Baylor GEMS pilot study. *Ethnicity and Disease, 13,* S30-S39.

Barrera, M., Glasgow, R. E., McKay, H. G., Boles, S. M., & Feil, E. G. (2002). Do Internet-based social support interventions change perceptions of social support?: An experimental trial of approaches for supporting diabetes self-management. *American Journal of Community Psychology, 30,* 637–654.

Clarke, G., Reid, E., Eubanks, D., O'Connor, E., DeBar, L. L., Kelleher, C., et al. (2002). Overcoming depression on the Internet (ODIN): A randomized controlled trial of an Internet depression skills intervention program. *Journal of Medical Internet Research, 4,* E14.

Edgar, L., Greenberg, A., & Remmer, J. (2002). Providing Internet lessons to oncology patients and family members: A shared project. *Psychooncology, 11,* 439–446.

Frenn, M., Malin, S., Bansal, N., Delgado, M., Greer, Y., Havice, M., et al. (2003). Addressing health disparities in middle school students' nutrition and exercise. *Journal of Community Health Nursing, 20,* 1–14.

Kemper, K. J., Amata-Kynvi, A., Sanghavi, D., Whelan, J. S., Dvorkin, L., Woo, A., et al. (2002). Randomized trial of an Internet curriculum on herbs and other dietary supplements for health care professionals. *Academic Medicine, 77,* 882–889.

Krishna, S., Francisco, B. D., Balas, E. A., Konig, P., Graff, G. R., & Madsen, R. W. (2003). Internet-enabled interactive multimedia asthma education program: A randomized trial. *Pediatrics, 111,* 503–510.

Kronick, J., Blake, C., Munoz, E., Heilbrunn, L., Dunikowski, L., & Milne, W. K. (2003). Improving online skills and knowledge. A randomized trial of teaching rural physicians to use online medical information. *Canadian Family Physician, 49,* 312–317.

Lenert, L., Munoz, R. F., Stoddard, J., Delucchi, K., Bansod, A., Skoczen, S., et al. (2003). Design and pilot evaluation of an Internet smoking cessation program. *Journal of the American Medical Informatics Association, 10,* 16–20.

Merion, R. M., Vinokur, A. D., Couper, M. P., Jones, E. G., Dong, Y., Wimsatt, M., et al. (2003). Internet-based intervention to promote organ donor registry participation and family notification. *Transplantation, 75,* 1175–1179.

Tate, D. F., Jackvony, E. H., & Wing, R. R. (2003). Effects of Internet behavioral counseling on weight loss in adults at risk for type 2 diabetes: A randomized trial. *Journal of the American Medical Association, 289,* 1833–1836.

White, H., McConnell, E., Clipp, E., Branch, L. G., Sloane, R. Pieper, C., et al. (2002). A randomized controlled trial of the psychosocial impact of providing Internet training and access to older adults. *Aging & Mental Health, 6,* 213–221.

Winzelberg, A. J., Classen, C., Alpers, G. W., Roberts, H., Koopman, C., Adam, R. E., et al. (2003). Evaluation of an Internet support group for women with primary breast cancer. *Cancer, 97,* 1164–1173.

Qualitative Research

Bette K. Idemoto

Qualitative nurse researchers are beginning to realize the breadth and depth of sources of potential study participants via the Internet. The review of literature presented below provides brief information on what qualitative nurse researchers have published to date using the Internet as a research methodology. Qualitative research using the Internet is in its infancy. In the future, expansion is likely. However, not all topics or methods of qualitative research are appropriate or desirable for Internet use.

1. WEB-BASED PATIENT-RELATED QUALITATIVE NURSING RESEARCH

Adler and Zarchin (2002) conducted a qualitative exploratory, descriptive study using purposive sampling methodology to examine the lived experience of pregnant women confined to home bed rest. Seven women confined to home bed rest for pre-term labor were interviewed over a 4-week timeframe via electronic mail using a series of questions developed by the researchers. Participants were recruited from a high-risk pregnancy Web site (four) and from a Northern California perinatal health maintenance organization (three). Privacy was assured throughout the study by setting up and maintaining a "closed, private communication system known as a 'listserv account'" (Adler & Zarchin, p. 420). The "virtual focus group process" identified categories of qualitative data for the lived experience of women with pre-term labor who were confined to bed rest. Three main categories emerged and included the effect of bed rest on participants' lives, the effect of bed rest on the women's relationships with others, and the virtual focus group as an online peer support group. Seven subcategories expanded the explanations of these categories.

    Dickerson, Flaig, and Kennedy (2000) investigated use of an electronic bulletin board by patients who received an implantable cardioverter defibrillator (ICD). Fifteen months of postings were collected from an electronic bulletin board between 1997 and 1998. The authors noted that at the time of the study, electronic bulletin boards were "considered public forums that anyone with access could read," (Dickerson et al., p. 250). All identifying information was deleted from the text. The research team protocol followed a phenomenological approach for discovering meanings in the posted messages. Four themes emerged from the sample of 75 online ICD persons who posted 469 interactions. The themes included: seeking and giving meaningful information, personal perspectives, storytelling, and supportive interacting. Themes were constructed into a therapeutic connection pattern that could then be used to develop online support for the ICD patients.

Giordano (1995) studied midlife women's health concerns via the Internet activity of 442 members of an online menopause discussion group who exchanged 3,892 communications from January to December 1994. Three topics emerged as significant to these women: health concerns, aging, and self-care. The major themes that surfaced within these topics were identity, autonomy, and generativity. Women were able to discuss experiences, knowledge, and perceptions as well as health care needs, uncertainty, and self-care practices openly and honestly.

Klemm, Hurst, Dearholt, and Trone (1999) examined whether the categories of responses for single gender were different from those where both genders participated in Internet cancer support groups (ICSG). Between September 15 and October 25, 1997, 325 consecutive ICSG postings were examined. Content analysis (line-by-line) produced four categories from the separate prostate, breast, and mixed ICSG: information giving/seeking (first in prostate cancer group), encouragement/support, personal opinion, and personal experience (first in breast cancer group). Activism was also a large category in the prostate only group; prayer was a major category in the mixed ICSG.

2. QUALITATIVE RESEARCH OF WEB-BASED INSTRUCTION

VandeVusse and Hanson (2000) evaluated online course discussions among graduate midwifery students and nursing faculty. Qualitative evaluation was the guiding framework for 604 double-spaced pages of online discussions that had been transcribed from sixteen students and two faculty members. Faculty communication that encouraged student participation in online discussions was coded. Categories and the analysis were reviewed by several faculty members who were not involved in the course. Six categories evolved that described faculty communication that facilitated active involvement by students: assistance with navigation, explaining expectations, clarifying the faculty role, stimulating critical thinking, sharing expertise, and providing encouragement.

REFERENCES

Adler, C. L., & Zarchin, Y. R. (2002). The "virtual focus group": Using the Internet to reach pregnant women on home bed rest. *Journal of Obstetric, Gynecologic, and Neonatal Nursing, 31,* 418–427.

Dickerson, S. S., Flaig, D. M., & Kennedy, M. C. (2000). Therapeutic connection: Help seeking on the Internet for persons with implantable cardioverter defibrillators. *Heart & Lung: Journal of Acute and Critical Care,* 29, 248–55.

Giordano, N. A. (1995). *An investigation of the health concerns of the menopause discussion group on Internet.* Dissertation abstracts International. Ed.D. Columbia University Teachers College.

Klemm, P., Hurst, M., Dearholt, S. L., & Trone, S. R. (1999). Cyber solace: Gender differences on Internet cancer support groups. *Computers in Nursing, 17,* 65–72.

VandeVusse, L., & Hanson, L. (2000). Evaluation of online course discussions. Faculty facilitation of active student learning. *Computers in Nursing, 18,* 181–8.

Appendix **2**

Web Resources for
Nursing Research

General Resources

Kristen S. Montgomery

This section highlights general research resources available on the Web relevant to nurses who conduct research. The sites detail resources to gain additional research knowledge, resources for funding, and pages that identify multiple resources. As more individuals become proficient in the mechanics of creating and maintaining Web sites, more sites are developed. Now, as more academics and researchers have embraced the phenomenon of Web hosting, more and more research and statistics resources have become available. Listed in this chapter are some of the most useful resources.

1. AMERICAN NURSES FOUNDATION (ANF) RESEARCH GRANTS PROGRAM

http://www.ana.org/anf

ANF is the national philanthropic organization that promotes the continued growth and development of nurses and services to advance the work of the nursing profession. The American Nurses Association sponsors the site. The most significant feature of this site is the information on the research grants program offered by ANF. Research grants are available in a variety of areas for both new and experienced researchers. Applications are available in January for a May 1 submission date. Candidates are notified of awards on October 1 of each year. Application packets can be downloaded from this site. Additional information is provided on the mission of ANF, its history, board of directors, and staff. The site is simple to use and organized in a clear manner. Text is provided in English at an average level.

2. GRADUATE RESEARCH ONLINE JOURNALS RESEARCH RESOURCES

http://www.graduateresearch.com/nsglinks.htm

Graduate Research Online Journals are edited and maintained by a doctoral candidate in nursing to provide a forum for graduate students to publish their research. This Web address is the research resources section of the journals' page. The resources include a list of links with relevance to nursing research. The following main sections are included: journal sites, research methods, statistics, conferences, nursing issues, nurse researcher database, funding information, nursing theorist sites, literature databases, writing and style manuals, online reference books, public policy and laws, research instruments, nursing organizations, standards and protocols, online nursing programs, healthcare metalinks and directories, and other nursing links. Some of these links are more directly related to research than others. Overall, the site is easy to use and is written at an average level in English. The Web site includes blinking advertisements as part of the medical banner exchange, which provides advertising posting to over 600 Web sites. An e-mail address is provided for the owner of the site and the site includes a search feature.

3. MCMASTER UNIVERSITY HEALTH SCIENCES LIBRARY GUIDE TO NURSING RESEARCH RESOURCES

http://www-hsl.mcmaster.ca/nursing/research.html

This Web site is a comprehensive list of Internet resources related to nursing research that was compiled by the librarians at McMaster University

Health Sciences Library. The resource list includes both qualitative and quantitative resources. Contact information is provided at the bottom of the page, as is the date of last update.

4. THE MIDWEST NURSING RESEARCH SOCIETY (MNRS)

http://www.mnrs.org

The Midwest Nursing Research Society is a membership organization that promotes the conduct of nursing research in the region and facilitates networking among nurse researchers. The site features the benefits of membership and information on the annual conference. Also included is information on publications, officers, governing board, committee membership, and research and grants information. The home page also contains contact information for the current president and the executive director of MNRS. The MNRS Web site is colorful and easy to use. The main categories of the site are all clearly listed on the home page. Text is presented at a simple level in English.

5. NATIONAL INSTITUTE OF NURSING RESEARCH (NINR)

http://www.nih.gov/ninr

The National Institute of Nursing Research (NINR) is the nursing research section of the National Institutes of Health (NIH). The site contains general information on NINR funding and activities and events sponsored by the institute. Descriptions of different types of NINR-funded awards and whom to contact within the institute are also available. The site includes the history of NINR, employment opportunities (both NINR and NIH), conferences, publications, speeches, a legislative activities section, and information on grants and funding. The "Research Program" section also includes separate sections for intramural and extramural research. The "Extramural" section includes links to the NIH, including training opportunities, CRISP (Computer Retrieval of Information on Scientific Projects—a searchable database of biomedical research projects funded by NIH) and NIH grants information and guides to grants and contracts. There is a small section on the collaborative activities between NINR and NIH. The application process is described along with current funded NINR grants, care centers, and institutional training programs. The NINR Web page also features areas of research opportunity for future fiscal years. The "Scientific Advances" section features highlights and outcomes of current nursing research and health information. The NINR Web page also features the strategic plan, with a mechanism to provide feedback to the NINR director. The NINR Web page is comprehensive, well organized, and easy to navigate. The color scheme enhances ease of use and organization. The text provides clear, succinct information at an average to high level in English.

6. RESEARCH! AMERICA

http://www.researchamerica.org

Research! America's mission is to make medical and health research a much higher national priority. It is a national nonprofit, membership-supported, public education and advocacy alliance, founded in 1989. The Web site provides general health research information for nurses, physicians, and other health care providers. Highlights include legislative links and an advocacy center. The home page features a brief description of the organization's mission, links for Research! America's polls, goals and initiatives of the organization, facts on medical research, and newsworthy events. The "Get Involved" section features information on how to contact Congress, including talking points and a mechanism to send a message to Congress via e-mail; the "Legislative Branch" section includes a mechanism to search for one's congressional representative by zip code. The "Executive and Judiciary Branch" section focuses on links to departments and agencies, and to searching the status of federal bills. There is also an option to search for information on federal bills by certain categories, for example, AIDS-related bills. Letter drafts, e-mail postcards, and a "Why Me?" section are also included. The "Medical Links" section is sorted by federal agencies, councils/think tanks, medical/science education, science policy, and international health policy. Lastly, there is a member's only section that is password protected. A site map is also available.

Colors on the site are well coordinated and feature red, white, and blue. Navigation through the site is easy. The design and layout of the site are frequently updated. Text is presented at an average level in English.

7. ROYAL COLLEGE OF NURSING'S RESEARCH AND DEVELOPMENT CO-ORDINATING CENTRE

http://www.man.ac.uk/rcn

The Royal College of Nursing (RCN) is the professional organization representing individual nurses in the United Kingdom. The RCN Research and Development Co-ordinating Centre houses the RCN Research Society, which has 11,500 members. One can link to a wide variety of different databases, including academic departments within the U. K. that offer a health-related course; the British Nursing Index, which contains references to over 220 nursing and allied health journals; cancer registries for Northern Ireland, East Anglia, Trent, Yorkshire, Europe, and international; CHAIN—Contact, Help, Advice and Information Network for evidence-based heath care; CINAHL; The Cochrane Collection; English National Board for Nursing, Midwifery, and Health Visiting; European Database on AIDS; evidence-based health resources; online nursing research journals; MEDLINE; National Co-ordinating Centre for Health Technology Assessment; National Research Registrar; National Health Services (NHS) Research and Development Outputs Database; RCN Library and Information Services Online Database; RD info, a digest of health-related funding opportunities; and REGARD—a search bibliographic database funded by the Economic and Social Research Council (ESRC). This is a fully interactive Web site. Job listings are also available. The RCN Research and Development Co-ordinating Centre provides high-quality information for nurses interested in the specific areas of expertise that are offered. While the information is good, the organization could be improved. As it stands, the information is somewhat disjointed. Text is provided in English at an average level.

8. THE ROYAL WINDSOR SOCIETY FOR NURSING RESEARCH

http://www.windsor.igs.net/~nhodgins

The society is a nonprofit association of nurse researchers living throughout the world and sharing an interest in nursing research; membership is free. This group is an Internet-based group, not related to any other professional nursing organization. The Web site contains information on nursing research conferences, centers of excellence, and international research institutions. In addition, the "Research Retrospective" section contains reports from history (such as "Childbed Fever in 19th Century Vienna"). There are also online workshops on topics such as literature search; and study design, analysis, reliability, and validity; with links to dictionaries (both multilingual and crosslingual). There is a section titled "Considerations in Study Design" which includes information on informed consent, treatment of gender groups, self-reporting, and much more. Finally, there is a nurse-to-nurse section that includes an online journal club with virtual peer review, newsgroups, and classified announcements. In the fun and games section, there is an opportunity to play Research Jeopardy. The Royal Windsor Society for Nursing Research Web site is well organized and colorful. The main sections are listed on the home page. The site offers many opportunities for discovering information. Text is provided at an average level in English.

9. SOUTHERN NURSING RESEARCH SOCIETY (SNRS)

http://www.snrs.org

The Southern Nursing Research Society Web site details resources that are available in the southern United States and includes information on membership in the society. The site also provides information on employment and training opportunities and the annual conference. Research interest groups, the Southern Online Journal of Nursing Research, newsletters, abstracts, and the membership directory can be accessed with membership. Overall, this is a very good site. All information is categorized on the home page for easy access. Organization is logical and clear. The site is in color, easy to navigate, and presented at an average level in English.

10. WORLD WIDE NURSE: NURSING RESEARCH FUNDING

http://www.wwnurse.com/nursing/research-funding.shtml

Highlights of the World Wide Nurse: Nursing Research Funding information Web page include a list of funding/grant resources with links to their respective pages, and a free nursing research chat room. A brief description of each section is provided. The Foundation Center, funding information from the Bureau of Health Professions' Grant Files, a funding opportunities database, grant and contact information from the National Institute of Health, the Fulbright Scholar Program, and the Robert Wood Johnson Foundation are featured. Advertising supports World Wide Nurse. Brian Short, a nurse based in Minnesota, produces it. Overall, this is a helpful Web site. The list of resources and the brief descriptions that accompany them are useful. Additionally, all of the information is provided in one location, which facilitates timely access. There is no apparent order to the listings, however. Also, the site features some blinking advertisements that are distracting.

Electronic Textbooks for Research

Kristen S. Montgomery

There are a variety of electronic textbooks available on the World Wide Web that are useful in research. Web-based electronic textbooks can be particularly useful for downloading to handheld computers that can be used in any research setting when they are free and thus easily accessible to all members of the research team via a simple Internet connection. Free and easy downloads are especially useful when team members are geographically distant. Wireless Internet systems are also useful to access Internet-based electronic textbooks when at a research site or geographically distant from the research team, as coinvestigators and consultants may be. Electronic textbooks can also be useful in online courses and continuing education (see chapters on CE and education for additional information).

Another benefit to the use of online electronic textbooks is that in many cases they are updated continuously, negating the need to purchase new print texts every few years. Most reputable publishers and organizations maintain their electronic books in this way. However, there are some electronic texts out there that are put online once and not updated. This should be readily apparent to the user by the lack of dates that provide the time of last update or when old dates are used. One should be suspicious of the quality and authenticity of the content if dates of publication and update are not available.

Textbooks that are available online should be held to the same scrutiny as other published works. For example, they need to be professionally published with accurate grammar and punctuation, authorship and affiliation must be clearly visible, and any sponsorship of the project or Web site should be noted. In addition, if the author has any conflicts or potential conflicts of interest, those should be freely disclosed to the user.

STATISTICAL BOOKS

Many online electronic books are available that address the appropriate use of statistics in research, basic principles of statistics, and analysis of data. The following section details some of these resources.

1. Concepts and Applications of Inferential Statistics

http://faculty.vassar.edu/lowry/webtext.html

This online electronic textbook is a free, full-text and occasionally interactive textbook on inferential statistics. This is the companion reference site for that statistical computation site VassarStats (http://faculty.vassar.edu/lowry/VassarStats.html) that is discussed below. Richard Lowry is the author of both sites. He is a professor of psychology at Vassar College in Poughkeepsie, New York. E-mail information is also available. The home page of Concepts and Applications of Inferential Statistics includes a "contents overview" and a table of contents of chapters that are divided into parts one and two. Topics include principles of measurement, distributions, correlation and regression, statistical significance, chi-square procedures, Analysis of Variance (ANOVA), and several appendices. The text is easy to follow and is available for printing.

2. VasserStats: Web Site for Statistical Computation

http://faculty.vassar.edu/lowry/VassarStats.html

VasserStats: Web Site for Statistical Computation is a useful and user-friendly tool to perform statistical computations. The site was developed by Richard Lowry, a professor at Vassar College. The home page of this site features a list of statistical computations that can be performed on the site. These include probabilities, distributions, proportions, correlation and regression, t-tests, ANOVA, ANCOVA, and miscellaneous others. The site also features clinical research calculators, a statistical tables calculator, a randomizer, a simple graph maker, note pad, pocket calculator, and portable document formatting (PDF) and Excel downloads. A site map is included.

3. Cyberstats

http://statistics.cyberk.com/splash/

This is the Web address for an electronic interactive textbook on statistics that was developed by Alexander Kugushev, President of Cybergnostics, Inc., an educational publisher that "delivers knowledge in electronic form." The book includes a complete online introductory statistics course with careful explanations and immediate feedback on practice problems. The book is useful in both distance and campus courses. Registration is required to use the site and students must pay a $30 registration fee. The site is free for institutions to use. The site has a free course management system that includes a test bank and a grade book that can automatically grade tests and quizzes. Six hundred interactive items are included that use real data in real world settings with an emphasis on data analysis and conceptual understanding. Analytic software (Webstat 3.0) provides computation, graphical data analysis, and processes Excel files. The software is adaptable based on individual preferences. The textbook and course is authored by 20 experienced statistics teachers and has been edited for consistency in language. The editor-in-chief of the project and the contributors are listed on the bottom of the home page along with their respective institutions. The site also includes a frequently-asked-questions section and a list of different uses for the Cyberstats program. The National Science Foundation funded development of the program.

4. StatSoft Electronic Textbook

http://www.statsoft.com/textbook/stathome.html

The StatSoft Electronic Textbook offers training in the understanding and application of statistics. The book was developed by the Research and Development department of StatSoft based on years of experience teaching undergraduate and graduate statistics courses. StatSoft is a company that makes high-performance statistical analysis and graphics software. The electronic textbook begins with an overview of statistics and then progresses to more complex content. Information is organized into learning modules. Each module is listed on the right side of the Web page for easy access. Some sample topics include elementary concepts, basic statistics, ANOVA/ Multiple Analyses of Variance (MANOVA), association rules, canonical analysis, classification trees, cluster analysis, data mining techniques, discriminant analysis, factor analysis, regression, partial least squares, power analysis, and quality control charts. Many other topics are included as this is a very comprehensive electronic textbook. The book also includes a statistical glossary, statistical advisor, distribution tables, and references. All information can be accessed for free.

RESEARCH BOOKS

In addition to statistics, several research methods books are available electronically via the Internet. Noted below are two excellent sites. General research information is less readily available than statistical material.

1.   Cornell University Research Methods Tutorial

http://trochim.human.cornell.edu/tutorial/TUTORIAL.htm

This Web resource is a list of exercises that are appropriate for an undergraduate or graduate student audience. A faculty member and graduate students at Cornell University developed the exercises. The site includes many topics which are separated into the following broad categories: foundations, sampling and external validity, measurement and construct validity, research design and internal validity, and data analysis and conclusion validity. The sections are easy to read and follow. A link is available to submit comments or questions. Because the exercises were developed by different individuals there are some differences in the quality and appearance of the exercises.

2.   Interactive Textbook on Clinical Symptom Research

http://www.neri.org/s1/tablecontents.htm

The Interactive Textbook on Clinical Symptom Research is a project of the New England Research Institute (NERI), a non-profit organization that focuses on clinically relevant research. NERI also produces various health-related publication materials such as booklets and videos. The U. S. Department of Health and Human Services, National Institute of Dental and Craniofacial Research funded this interactive textbook project. A link is available to send questions or comments. Detailed information on the two main physician editors is also available. Information about individual chapter authors is found at the beginning of each chapter. Most of the authors are physicians, however, a few are from other disciplines including nursing.

The Interactive Textbook on Clinical Symptom Research is easy to read and very user-friendly. The home page lists chapter topics and authors with their credentials and clinical affiliations. A link to the home page can be found at the top of each page. There is also a "go to" feature that lets the user select a topic from a menu bar. The textbook is very comprehensive.

Chapter topics include:

- The Design of Clinical Trials for Treatment of Pain
- Development of a Clinical Trial
- Methods for Clinical Research in Constipation
- The Psychology of Patient Decision-Making
- Delirium Research Questions
- Within Patient Studies: Cross-Over Trials and n-of-1 Studies
- Selected Qualitative Methods
- Statistical Models for Prognostication
- Fatigue
- Evaluating Health Care Systems for Improving Symptom Management
- Chemotherapy Related Nausea and Vomiting
- Clinical Economics
- Learning from Quality Improvement in Health Care Systems
- Tools for Decision-Making
- Challenges to the Study of Insomnia and Sleep Loss, and
- Somatization and Symptom Evaluation.

The following topics are noted to be in preparation:

- dyspnea
- oral mucositis
- pain as a model of neurobiology of symptoms

- epidemiology of symptoms in advanced illness
- hospice use
- secondary analysis of large survey databases
- desirability of outcome states
- dry mouth
- clinical trials in temporomandibular disorders (TMD)
- TMD: human experimental models, and
- epidemiology of TMD

COMPREHENSIVE LISTS OF STATISTICAL AND RESEARCH RESOURCES

Below are two Web sites that each address a comprehensive list of resources that may be useful to researchers.

- Fayetteville State University, Charles W. Chesnutt Library http://wwwlib.uncfsu.edu/reference/quantitative_research_web-sites.htm

This listing includes topics that are categorized as government and associations, tests and measurement, calculators online, a select list of journals, research methods, statistical guides, and human subjects research information.

- Online Statistical Textbooks and Courses: http://www.uni-koeln. delthemen/statistik/onlinebooks.html

SUMMARY

A variety of research resources exist as electronic textbooks on the World Wide Web. Nurse researchers are encouraged to explore these resources as they offer the benefits of convenience and low cost or free use. Many resources exist for statistical knowledge and computation. Fewer resources exist for research methodologies. Nurse researchers are cautioned to carefully evaluate any online electronic textbook in the same manner they would a print book.

Nursing Theory

Lucinda Farina, Joyce J. Fitzpatrick, and Kristen S. Montgomery

Nursing theory is an integral part of the development of the scientific enterprise. Nursing theory is used as a guide to education, practice, and research. There are three basic levels of theory addressed in the nursing literature: grand, middle range, and practice level. Grand theory articulates the philosophical beliefs and goals of the profession; middle range theory includes testable hypotheses; practice level theory addresses practice issues and, through an inductive process, builds theory. As practicing nurses search for understanding of why we do what we do as nurses, nursing theory offers explanation and definition of who we are and what we do. Yet, there are few Web sites that detail specific nursing theories; most of the Web sites available are devoted to grand theories. The Web sites chosen for review were selected for their potential to assist the practicing nurse in identifying nursing theories, including middle range and grand theories.

1. THE COMFORT LINE

http://www.uakron.edu/comfort/

This seven-page Web site is devoted to describing and explaining middle range theory developed by Kathy Kolcaba, PhD, RN, C, nursing faculty at the University of Akron. The Comfort Theory and its use for practice and research is well-articulated and diagrammed for professional caregivers and researchers. Healthcare administrators will be interested in how the Comfort Theory impacts institutional integrity. Dr. Kolcaba's telephone number and e-mail address are listed on the Web page and interested parties are encouraged to contact her with questions for either practice or research.

Kolcaba has created sections within the Web page to address specific applications of the Comfort Theory to practice and to research. The research instrument, the General Comfort Questionnaire, is included on the Web page. References are provided to Kolcaba's work and to pertinent works of other authors. The section on development of the Comfort Theory discusses the grand theories that guided the development of the theory. Easy to navigate, recently updated, and available in English only, this Web site is an excellent source for nurses learning to build middle range theory because the process of theory building is clearly modeled.

2. NURSES.INFO

http://www.nurses.info

Nurses.info is a very comprehensive Web site that includes information on nursing theory. The site was designed specifically for nurses and is managed by John Turner, RN. The site is new, first being published on May 17, 2003, and added to major search engines in July 2003. The creators have the ambitious goal of providing the most extensive and diverse nursing site on the Internet. So far, they are doing a good job. The nursing theorists list is quite comprehensive and includes the well-known theorists as well as some of the lesser-known theorists. The site is easy to use and is clearly organized. The site is only available in English.

3. NURSESCRIBE

http://www.enursescribe.com/nurse_theorists.htm

NurseScribe is a Web site that provides multiple clinical and professional resources for nurses. A list of twenty contemporary U. S. theorists, Nightingale, and links to sites about their work are included as one of the resources offered. The site, which is maintained by Becky Sisk, PhD, RN, is available in English only. The site has been recently updated, presents information clearly, and is easy to navigate. Most importantly, the links worked when tested. Nurse theorists are categorized clearly according to their theories, and include early nurse theorists such as Peplau and Henderson, well-known grand theorists, and middle range theorists. Also included are links to University-based theory pages that list nursing theorists and links to individual Web pages. The only negative aspects of this Web site are the many advertisements and the layout of the Web page, which includes the middle third of the page as text with multiple advertisements on each side. Because the nursing theory text in the middle is narrow, the reader must scroll down frequently to get to the content.

4. THE NURSING THEORY PAGE

http://www.sandiego.edu/nursing/theory/#Theories

This site lists 24 nursing theorists and frequently provides multiple links for an individual theorist. Also included on this Web site are links to other nursing theory list sites, nursing theory conferences, literature search tips located under "Dear Student," resources in French and English, and teaching tools. A list of links to related resources includes nursing theorists not included on the main list. Why this distinction has been made is not identified on the Web site.

This collaborative effort by an international group was begun in 1996 and identifies itself as always a work in progress. Ann M. Mayo, RN, DNSc, who is a member of the faculty at the University of San Diego, maintains the site. The site was recently updated. This easily navigated site provides access to individual authors via e-mail addresses found under "About this group project." Feedback and contributions by site visitors are encouraged.

5. WATSON'S THEORY OF HUMAN CARING

http://www2.uchsc.edu/son/caring/content/default.asp

The purpose of this Web site is to educate nurses and other caregivers about Watson's Theory of Human Caring. The three pages of the Web site are written by Jean Watson, PhD, RN, FAAN, professor of nursing at the University of Colorado and director of the Center for Human Caring, in a style that is easy for any reader to comprehend. The site is well maintained by the Center for Human Caring executive director Karen Holland. Telephone number, e-mail, and fax for Watson and Holland are listed on the site. Information provided on this easily navigated Web site is current and accurate. It is available only in English. The theory of caring, its assumptions and definitions are clearly explained. A lengthy list of publications is provided to assist interested parties in studying Watson's theory.

Other Theories Used by Nurses

Kristen S. Montgomery

While the use of nursing theory is necessary to build nursing science and to distinguish nursing as a distinct discipline, nurses sometimes find it useful to use nursing theories in conjunction with theories developed by other similar disciplines. Therefore, several useful Web sites that provide links to theories developed by other disciplines are provided for nurses who may be interested in using them in their own work. Both of the sites listed below are sites that list numerous links to other sites (like a depository) rather than providing any theoretical information themselves.

1. EXPLORATIONS IN LEARNING AND INSTRUCTION: THE THEORY INTO PRACTICE DATABASE

http://tip.psychology.org

Explorations in Learning and Instruction: The Theory Into Practice Database (TIP) is a tool intended to make learning and instructional theory more accessible to educators. The database contains brief summaries of 50 major theories that are relevant to learning and instruction. The site was developed by Greg Kearsley and an e-mail address and home Web page are provided for additional information. Dr. Kearsley is an independent consultant who designs, develops, and teaches online courses. He has held multiple faculty positions and positions in the private section. Permission is granted to use the materials in educational and other non-commercial purposes. "Learning" is defined rather broadly. Some theories included in this database that are particularly relevant to nurse researchers include: Constructivist Theory (J. Brunner), Gestalt Theory (M. Wertheimer), Information Processing Theory (G. A. Miller), Operant Conditioning (B. F. Skinner), Social Development (L. Vygotsky), and Social Learning Theory (A. Bandura). Each description includes an overview, scope/application, examples, principles, and reference material. Relationships between theories are identified by highlighted text within articles. Theories were selected for inclusion in the database based on that they are published in the English language and that they address some aspect of human learning and instruction. The authors of the Web site note that theories that focus on animal learning, neuropsychology, learning disabilities, or teaching strategies are excluded as are theories of learning that have limited scientific support or are primarily philosophical in nature. Theories are addressed in their most updated form only; thus the database is most useful for doing a brief review of theories for potential use or applicability. Links to many of the original articles are provided for those interested in learning more history. The Web page is only available in English and is easy to navigate. The text is clear and concise.

2. HEALTH BEHAVIOR CHANGE: THEORIES AND MODELS

http://www.med.usf.edu/~kmbrown/hlth_beh_models.htm

The Health Behavior Change Web site is a list of theories and models that related to the health behavior change. The Web site was developed and is maintained by the University of South Florida Medical School Department of Community and Family Health. This Web page includes links to 10 different theories and models that are categorized by: models of individual health behavior, models of interpersonal behavior, and an "other" category. Theories and models particularly relevant to nursing include: The Health Belief Model, Theoretical Model/Stages of Change, Theory of Reasoned Action/Theory of Planned Behavior, Health Locus of Control, Social Cognitive Theory, PRECEDE/PROCEED, Ecological Models, and Attribution Theory. Some links provide detailed information and other only offer brief descriptions. The Web page was developed by Kelli McCormack Brown; however, the links have not been updated since 1999. Permission is granted to link to this page if desired. The site is only available in English and is easy to use.

Writing Resources

Kristen S. Montgomery

Writing is one of the essential tools for communication among human beings. Nurse researchers must excel in writing if they are to be successful researchers. From the very beginning of a research idea, researchers must be able to communicate that idea to others. While oral conversation often occurs in an informal situation, generally more formal communications are written and then perhaps followed up with a telephone conversation. Thus, nurse researchers need to have skills in writing. This review of Web resources includes general writing resources with information on the basics of writing, including grammar and punctuation, and more advanced writing resources that include information on proposal development and disseminating research results through publication in scholarly journals.

1. 11 RULES OF WRITING

http://www.junketstudies.com/rulesofw/

11 Rules of Writing is a concise guide to the most commonly violated rules of writing, grammar, and punctuation. The 11 rules are listed; clicking on one of the rules provides further information and examples of correct and incorrect use. The site is intended for all audiences to aid in learning and refining writing skills. The Web site is sponsored by Junket Studies Tutoring, a private tutoring company for elementary to college level, located in northern New Jersey. Examples, references to find information, and explanations are offered on the site. There is also a glossary to look up grammatical terms. A frequently-asked-questions section and word-of-the-day are other key features of this site. There is also a teacher's section that some individuals might find helpful. An e-mail address is provided for questions. Content is provided at an average to high level in English.

2. AMERICAN PSYCHOLOGICAL ASSOCIATION (APA) ONLINE—APASTYLE.ORG

http://www.apastyle.org

APA Style.org is a related link of the American Psychological Association (APA). This site features information on the APA style guidelines and related products that are for sale online. Helpful books that are available for purchase include *Displaying Your Findings* and *The Publication Manual.* Several workbooks are also featured: *Mastering APA Style* and

Instructor's Manual for Mastering APA Style. A list of the electronic products available through APA is also included. The site features a list of "quick tips" related to APA style that is useful for quickly looking up information on APA style. Contact information is provided for the organization and there is a service available that will send free e-mail updates to persons who chose to enter their e-mail address. The site also features information about APA's *E-reference guide* and *APA Style-Helper,* the companion to APA's popular *Publication Manual.* Finally, there is information on the ethics of publishing, ordering materials online, and a search feature.

3. ASIAN INSTITUTE OF TECHNOLOGY EXTENSION CENTER LANGUAGE CENTER'S WRITING UP RESEARCH

http://www.clet.ait.ac.th/el21open.htm

This Web site is a writing resource that is sponsored by the Asian Institute of Technology (AIT). AIT is an international graduate institution of higher learning with a mission to develop highly qualified and committed professionals who will play a leading role in the sustainable development of the region and its integration into the global economy. The site is written in English and is designed to be used for independent learning. Content is directed toward master's and other students involved in research projects. The site addresses the main components of a proposal and thesis and discusses the function of the major elements. There is no fee or registration required to use this site. The site was developed in 1997–1998 and has been updated regularly since its inception. A link is provided to submit comments or suggestions. The Web site is divided into two main sections including contents of the site and how to use the site. The "Contents" section includes information on the following topics: abstract, introduction, literature review, methodology (includes information on verb tenses and use of active and passive voice), results, discussion, and conclusion. All sections are succinct and presented clearly. The Web site also includes sections on the basics of good writing, how to reference, and useful writing links. References for the Web site content are also provided. Contact information in Thailand is provided along with an e-mail address. The language of the site is written in a clear and simple way that is ideal for students who may not speak English as their first language.

4. GUIDE FOR WRITING A FUNDING PROPOSAL

http://www.learnerassociates.net/proposal

The purpose of this Web site is to provide detailed information and examples to individuals working on research proposals that will be submitted to organizations for funding. S. Joseph Levine, PhD of Michigan State University (MSU), wrote this funding guide. E-mail address and the date of last update are provided. There are also links to "Guide for Writing and Presenting Your Thesis or Dissertation" and "Selection of Books to Help With the Preparation of a Funding Proposal." The main sections of the Web site include sections of a proposal: title, project overview, background/statement of problem, project detail, available resources, needed resources, evaluation plan, and appendices. One can click on "writing hints" or "example" to obtain the information in a way that is most useful to one's individual learning needs. One can also view an entire proposal sample or all of the writing hints by clicking on a link at the bottom of the page. A Portable Document Format (PDF) version is also available for printing. The Web site is easy to use and is clearly written. The only identified weakness of the site is that there is no information given on the success of individuals who have used these tips in obtaining funding nor is there any information about the funding history of the author. However, looking at the MSU home Web page, it is revealed that the author of this Web site is a full professor.

5. INDISPENSABLE WRITING RESOURCES

http://www.quintcareers.com/writing

Indispensable Writing Resources is a general writing Web site, sponsored by Quintcareers.com. Main sections of content include reference materials (a list of quality print resources), writing style guides (a list of general and specific subjects), and links to writing resources available on the Internet. There is also information on the importance of good writing skills. While the site is geared toward college students, it is useful to nurses as a general writing reference. Content is presented in English at an average level.

6. UNIFORM REQUIREMENTS FOR MANUSCRIPTS SUBMITTED TO BIOMEDICAL JOURNALS

http://www.icmje.org/

This Web site details the manuscript guidelines developed by the International Committee of Medical Journal Editors (ICMJE) who wanted to have uniform requirements for all journals that adhered to certain principles. These editors and their respective affiliations are noted at the end of the homepage. The date content was last updated is available on the site. The Web site also includes a section titled: "Publication Ethics: Sponsorship, Authorship, and Accountability." The main content categories available on this site are: redundant publication, secondary publication, privacy, reporting guidelines, manuscripts, authorship, and reference styles. These topics are identified as "things to consider before publication" and are listed in the upper-left-hand corner of the home page. Immediately below these topics are a list of statements regarding topics of interest to writers and editors. These include: peer review, editorial freedom, conflict of interest, industry support, corrections and retractions, confidentiality, journals and media, Internet, advertising, supplements, correspondence columns, and competing manuscripts. Another section addresses information about the ICMJE and lists the journals that adhere to the ICMJE Uniform Requirements. Contact information is provided for inquires related to the Uniform Requirements or the ICMJE.

7. UNIVERSITY OF WISCONSIN AT MADISON GRANTS INFORMATION CENTER

http://www.library.wisc.edu/libraries/Memorial/grants/proposal.htm

This Web address goes to a link at the University of Wisconsin library that lists proposal writing resources available on the Internet. This is a very comprehensive list that includes 25 different sites. Contact information is provided for the librarian who developed and maintains the list. A last-modified date is included. The sites included in this list address different perspectives and focus on different sections of the proposal. The site is easy to use and is clearly written in English.

Index

in research
    advantages of, 54–55
    disadvantages of, 55–56
    overview of, 53–54
    security, 128
    software, 122, 124
    use of, generally, 52–53, 55
PhD programs, online
    course management system
        (CMS), 172–175
    curriculum, 172
    electronic dissertations, 175–176
    evaluation of, 176–177
    historical perspectives, 171–175
    research skills development, 176
Planning phase, 10–15
Platform selection, 122–123
Portable disks, 125
Portable document format (PDF), con-
    version to, 26, 31–32, 226
Premier, 22
Principal Investigator (PI), functions of,
    138
Printing, security strategies, 132
Privacy issues, 112–113
Private domain, 108–109, 116
Professional organizations, 22
Program announcements (PA), 94
Programming languages, 70–71
Proposals, writing guidelines, 92,
    97–102
ProQuest, 176
Protection of Human Subjects of Bio-
    medical and Behavioral
    Research, 106
Prototype collaboratories, 62–63
Proximity operators, 15
Proxy server, 33
PSYCHInfo, 4, 11
Psychometrics, 101
Public domain, 108–109, 116
PubMed
    characteristics of, generally, 9–11, 13
    online journal directory, 14
    searching tips, 13–14
    Tutorial, 148, 153

PubMed Central (PMC), 13

QSR International, 5
Qualitative analysis software, 5
Qualitative research projects
    nursing research, 204–205
    web-based instruction, 205
Quality improvement, 20

Racial identity, 106–107
Randomization, 84
Reading skills development, research
    education, 148–149
Regulations/legislation, 50, 56, 76–77,
    97, 106–107, 163
Relational databases, 121–122
Reliability, 86, 98
Removable disks, 125
Request for Application (RFA), 94
Request for Proposals (RFPs), 94
Research! America, 210
Research assistants (RAs), 181
Research collaboratories
    benefits of, 66
    defined, 57–59
    examples of, 60–61
    health care, 61–63
    psychosocial issues, 65
    requirements, 63–65
Research methods
    intervention research, 43
    qualitative, 43–44
    survey research, 41–43, 69–77
Research projects, samples
    internet-based intervention,
        198–202
    qualitative research, 203–205
    survey research, 193–197
Research subjects
    profile of, 109–110
    protection of, 105–107
    recruitment, 47–51, 84–85
    sampling, 48–49, 75, 82–84
Research topic assessment
    controlled vocabulary, 10
    free text vocabulary, 9

Sub-notebook computers, 124
Supportive learning theory, 87
Survey modalities, 195–196
Survey research
advantages of, 73–74, 77–78
components of, 41–43
data analysis, 77
historical perspective, 70
methodology, 75–77
programming languages, 70–71
questionnaire, 71–73
sample projects, 193–197
SurveyWiz, 72
Susan Komen Breast Cancer Foundation, 95–96
Synchronous interaction, 110
Systems theory, 87

Tablet PCs, 124
Teaching research online
continuing education, 178–181
graduate courses, 157–169
PhD programs, 171–177
research utilization challenges, 182–191
undergraduate research education, 145–153
Teaching strategies, generally
graduate research courses, 163–164
undergraduate research education, 150–153
Technology, Education, and Copyright Harmonization (TEACH) Act, 163
Technology Assessment Model, 87–88
TELEform 8.2, 121
The Comfort Line, 219–220
Theories, web resources for, 222–223
Theory into Practice (TIP) database, 222–223
Trojan horses, 133–134, 137
Troubleshooting, 16
Truncation, 15–16
Tuskegee Syphilis Study, 105–106, 151

Tutorials, 16–18, 148, 153, 216

UMI ProQuest Digital Dissertations, 26–27, 30, 34, 36
Undergraduate research education
critical thinking skills, 145–146
critiquing research, 145–146, 149–150
evidence-based practice, 146–147
literature searching, 147–148
reading and comprehending research, 148–149
resources, 153
teaching strategies, 150–153
United States Copyright Office Library of Congress, 35
U.S. Department of Health and Human Services, Office of Civil Rights, 56
U.S. Government Healthcare Databases, 11, 13–14
Universal serial bus (USB), 124, 137
University Health-System Consortium (UHC), 22
University of San Diego, nursing theory page, 221
University of Wisconsin-Madison, Grants Information Center, 227
Unix, 123

Validity, 86, 98
VasserStats, 214–215
Video conferencing, 64
Video graphics array (VGA), 124
Virtual nuclear magnetic resonance (NMR), 60
Virtual Nursing College, 62–63
Virtual private network (VPN) software, 126, 128
Viruses
damage from, 101, 131–133
types of, 130
Vocabulary, types of, 9–10
Voluntariness, 114
Voluntary Hospitals of America (VHA), 22

Springer Publishing Company

Research in Nursing and Health
Second Edition
Understanding and Using Quantitative and Qualitative Methods

Carol Noll Hoskins, PhD, RN, FAAN

Carla Mariano, EdD, RN, HNC, FAAIM

This updated new edition offers the reader a step-by-step guide to conducting research and to understanding the research studies done by others. It describes both quantitative and qualitative investigations. The book is written in outline format, for quick reference. An important feature of the new edition is an extensive listing of online databases and knowledge resources. Graduate students and nurse researchers will find this an easily accessible source of valuable information.

Partial Contents:

- Introduction to Research, *C. Hoskins & C. Mariano*
- The Research Question, *C. Hoskins & C. Mariano*
- A Review of the Literature Using Online & Print Sources, *B. Carty et al.*
- Theoretical and Conceptual Frameworks, *C. Hoskins & C. Mariano*
- Research Designs, *C. Hoskins & C. Mariano*
- Sampling Methods: Basic Issues and Concepts, *C. Mariano & J. Giacquinta*
- Principles of Measurement, *C. Hoskins & H. Feldman*
- Development of Quantitative Measures, *C. Hoskins*
- Data Analysis and Interpretation, *C. Hoskins & C. Mariano*
- Product of the Inquiry: The Research Report, *C. Hoskins & C. Mariano*
- Guide to Critique of Quantitative Research—with Examples and Practice Studies, *C. Hoskins*
- Guide to Critique of Qualitative Research–with Examples and Practice Studies, *C. Mariano*
- Appendices: Suggested Guide for Abstracting Research Studies; Guide to Critique of Philosophical Research; Issues of Control and Validity: Quantitative Studies; Testing Hypotheses with an Exemplar Study: Statistical Significance, Error, Directionality, and Power

2004   200pp   0-8261-1616-7   softcover

11 West 42nd Street, New York, NY 10036-8002 • **Fax: 212-941-7842**
Order Toll-Free: 877-687-7476 • **Order On-line: www.springerpub.com**

Springer Publishing Company

Annual Review of 〜NEW〜
Nursing Research, *Volume 22*

Eliminating Health Disparities Among Racial and Ethnic Minorities in the United States

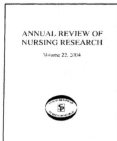

Joyce Fitzpatrick, PhD, RN, FAAN
Editor-in-Chief

Antonia M. Villarruel, PhD, RN, FAAN
Cornelia P. Porter, PhD, RN, FAAN
Volume Editors

This volume critically examines the research base on health disparities among racial and ethnic minorities in order to inform and advance nursing science in this area. It was created with the support and input of the National Coalition of Ethnic Minority Nurse Associations, and incorporates the expertise of distinguished minority nurse researchers. The major groups discussed include African-American, Hispanic, American Indian/Alaska Native, and Asian/Pacific. Differences in environment; access, utilization, and quality of care; and health status are addressed, as well as strengths of minority groups in promoting health and managing illness within current social and political contexts.

Partial Contents:
Part I: Factors Contributing to Health Disparities • Structural and Racial Barriers to Healthcare, *L. Bolton, J. Giger and C. Georges* • Language Barriers and Access to Care, *S. Yeo*

Part II: Special Populations • Health Disparities among Men from Racial and Ethnic Minority Populations, *C. Dallas and L. Burton* • African American and Asian American Elders: An Ethnogeriatric Perspective, *M. McBride and D. Lewis*

Part III: Special Conditions • Cancer among and between United States Ethnic and Racial Minority Populations, *S. Underwood et al.*

Part IV: Intervention Approaches for Racial and Ethnic Minority Populations • Utilization of Complementary and Alternative Medicine Among Racial and Ethnic Minority Populations, *R. Struthers and L. Nichols*

2004   368pp   0-8261-4134-X   hardcover

11 West 42nd Street, New York, NY 10036-8002 • Fax: 212-941-7842
Order Toll-Free: 877-687-7476 • Order On-line: www.springerpub.com